Book VALUES

connection
responsibility
economical
practical
access
life
fairness
sustainability
empowerment
nutrition
education
interaction
maximising potential
health
modelling
wholefood
longevity
seasonality
consistency
appreciation
equity
realistic
credibility

AF583579

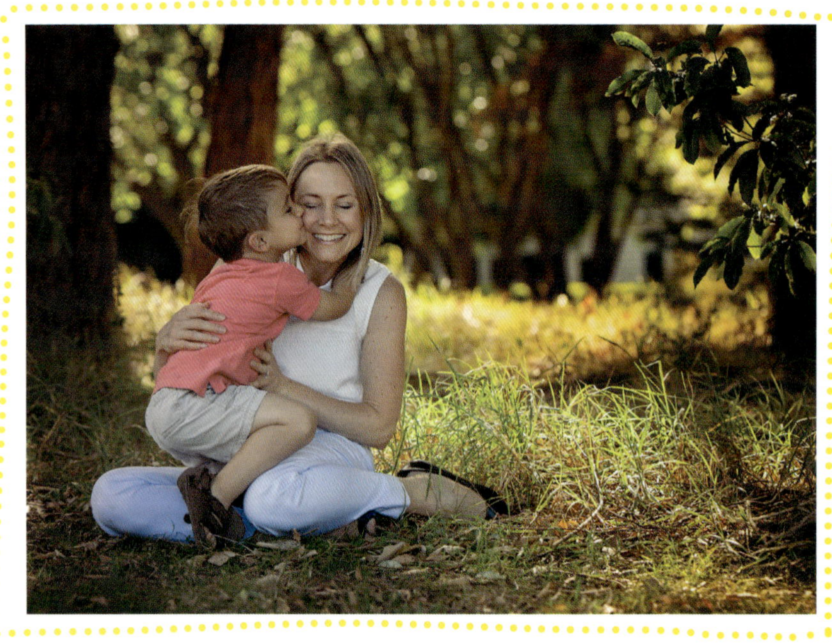

About BITE NUTRITION and the author

Bite Nutrition was created to offer practical, simple, beautiful books and tools to help carers, parents and educators get their children interested in their health and nutrition.

After years of working with adults as a Dietitian, the founder and author, Tanya Nagy decided she wanted to focus on educating humans when they were much younger; with no doubt that so much of who we are as adults is from our very early years of life. Hence, the series "Feeding Growing Humans Beautiful Yummy Food" was created. To help towards introducing the best foods for growth and long term health and giving our children the best start we can.

A mother of 3 beautiful little ones, Tanya is keen to contribute and have a positive impact on the world. She believes we should all be more personally responsible for our behaviors and impact on the environment; with special consideration to sustainability, respect, kindness and paying it forward.

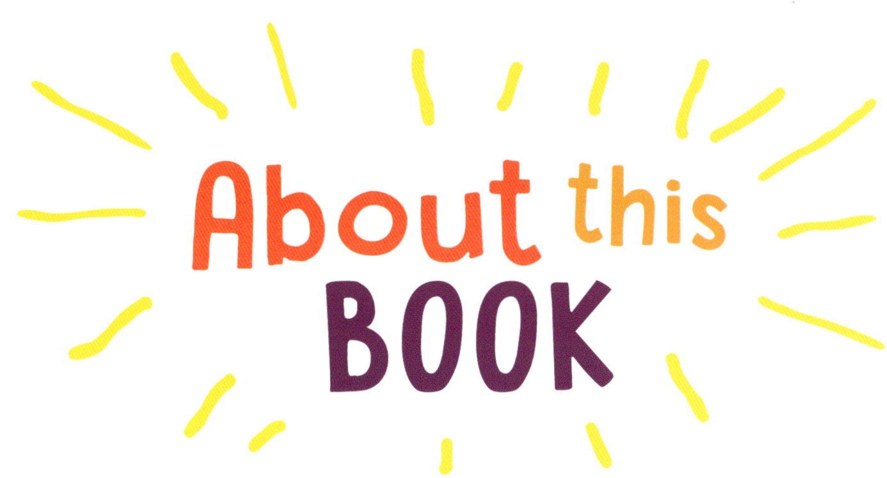

About this BOOK

You have this book because someone really **CARES** for you.
So, who gave you this book?

They want you to learn how to make **better choices** in the food you eat.

They want you to live a **LONG and HEALTHY Life** and be the **best that you can be.**

You are growing and as part of growing, your body needs helpful foods; foods that help you grow in a **healthy** way.

Sometimes what your body "needs" to be healthy and what you "want" because it tastes good can be different. Let's think of some examples of that.

Can YOU think of any?

This book is to show you real to life pictures of important foods that you need to learn about. It also tells you:

1 What "season" the food is best.

2 How the food grows.

3 How each food is HELPFUL to your body.

4 How much of each food you should eat each time and over the day.

5 A recipe for each food and some tips on how to shop for it and store it

Have fun learning about these **Beautiful Yummy Foods!** Then each day, let's try to choose what your body needs, most of the time!

What older readers SHOULD KNOW

This book is **NOT** designed to be an encyclopaedia of vegetables. It has only some of the vegetables we have to choose from. The vegetables chosen, were chosen because they are one or a few of these following points:

1. Rich in **nutrition** (nutrient dense).
2. **Accessible** (i.e. volume, cost, found in most markets).
3. Can be used easily as **lunchbox/on the go** options.

want a vegetable in the next book version? contact us @

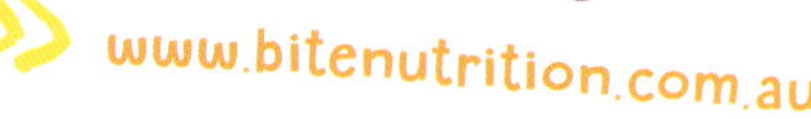

When you read to your younger learner, keep these things in mind.

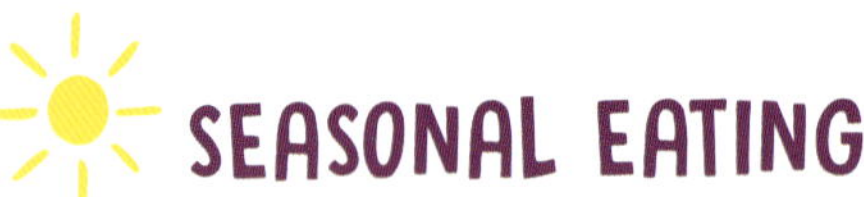

Choosing food in season is better for your health, the environment and your budget! Vitamins and minerals are at their highest in content in season. Also, the vitamins and minerals the foods in season have are those that your body needs the most at that time of year.

SEASONS KEY:

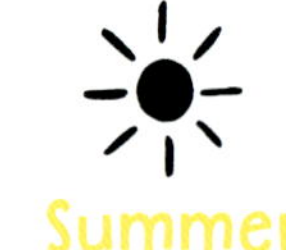

Summer
December, January, February

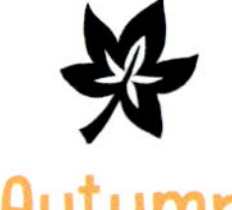

Autumn
March, April, May

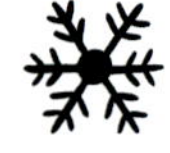

Winter
June, July, August

Spring
September, October, November

HOW FOOD IS GROWN

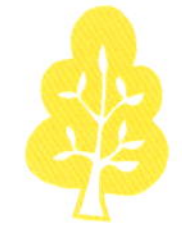

"Where does food come from?" *The shop?* It is important our children understand the food cycle and value the work our farmers do. Food takes a lot of effort to produce and learning about this will help them appreciate food more and hopefully, slowly, discourage them from wasting food!

SERVES AND VARIETY

Variety of food is so important for health. Too much of any food, even "healthy" food, is not helpful. Look at the colours in a rainbow and try to eat lots of colours, in foods, each day. There are many colours of vegetables, so try to eat at least 3 different colours each day in the right (total) serve size.

SERVES

Adults are recommended to have 5-6 serves of vegetables **every day**.
Children's needs are less:

1-2 yrs = 2-3 serves of vege

2-3 yrs = 2 ½ serves of vege

4-8 yrs = 4 ½ serves of vege

9-11+ yrs = 5 serves of vege.

FRESH/FROZEN/CANNED/DRIED/BLENDED

What is best!? **Fresh in season is best** where you can. Next best is snap frozen, canned, blended then dried. Whole fresh vegetables, skin on where possible, is always going to be better for you.

VITAMINS AND MINERALS—TRYING TO KEEP THEM

- Always wash your vegetables before preparing them.
- Do not peel your vegetables if you can avoid it; unless the skin is not edible. You can eat most vegetables skin. The skin has lots of great fibre to help your tummy and there are lots of vitamins just under the skin you may peel away.
- Try not to chop your vegetables too much. The vitamins inside break very easily and lots of chopping is not helpful in keeping the vitamins.
- As soon as you start to heat vegetables, the vitamins and minerals inside will start to disappear. Do not boil vegetables in water, as the vitamins leave the vegetable and go into the water and are destroyed. Vegetables are best crisp by lightly steaming them or rapid blanching. But the longer the vegetable stays hot, the more nutrition is lost through heat.

B1

THE IMPORTANCE OF WATER

An average of 70% of your body is water. Plain, clean water helps your body; including getting oxygen to your brain so you can think, concentrate, learn and be at your full potential. Other fluids are not as helpful. More water please!!!

BEES

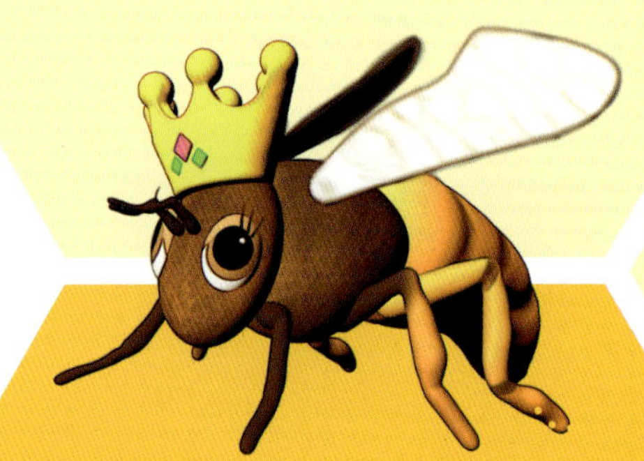

The **QUEEN BEE** can live up to 7 years though, but that is because the bees don't let her do any work other than lay eggs.

Honey is precious! A worker bee only lives for 6 weeks in season and in that time, she will make 1⁄12th of a teaspoon of honey.

Please learn more about bees and take care of them. They are very **precious**.

How does a bee make honey? She sucks nectar from the centre of flowers and stores it in a separate container inside of her. Then she gets back to the hive and either puts it into the hexagon storage cells straight away, or she passes it to other bees who work to get the water out of the nectar so it becomes **HONEY**!

Bees are **very smart**! In many ways. But their hives hexagon shapes tells you how smart they are. It's the strongest shape, that take the least amount of wax to create and allows the most amount of honey and eggs to be stored in it. Very smart indeed.

You will find Orla on the pages where she is needed to create the vegetable and where she helps the size and amount of the vegetable a plant grows.

How to READ this BOOK

TODDLERS

1. Look at the pictures
2. Learn to recognize the vegetables
3. Look for Orla

PRESCHOOLERS

1. Learn which season its best
2. Learn where it grows
3. Learn how the food can help you
4. Learn what a serve size is
5. Talk about eating fresh vegetables each day

SCHOOL KIDS

1. Pick one vegetable each week
2. Look at the recipe and go shopping for it
3. Practice how to choose and store the vegetable
4. Then prepare the recipe and eat!

YOU CAN ALSO...

1. Learn how important bees are to our environment
2. Learn the book values and add some of your own
3. Do the quiz at the back!

CAPSICUM

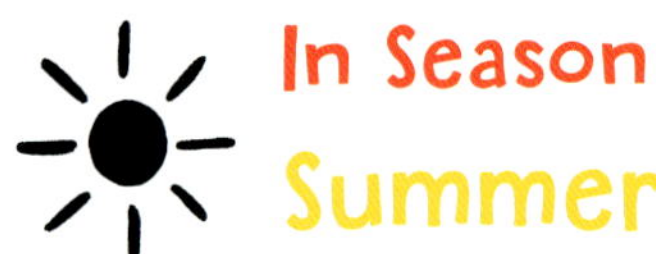

In Season

Summer

Grows How?

On vines

A Serve

1 cup

Good For Your

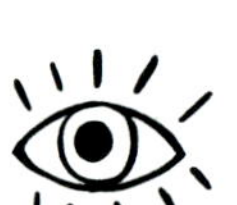

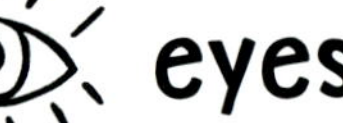

eyes

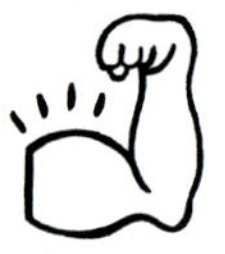

strength

heart

Recipe

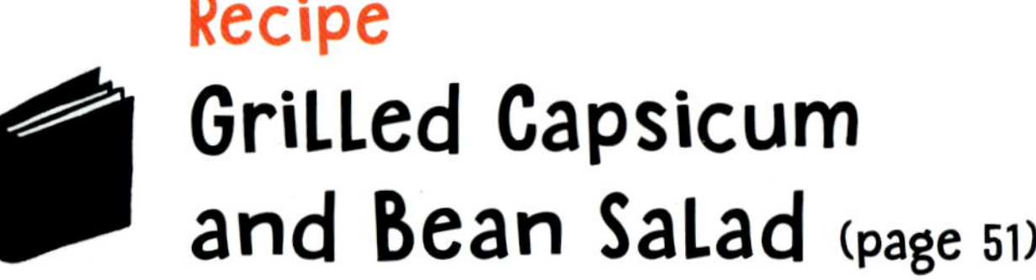

Grilled Capsicum and Bean Salad (page 51)

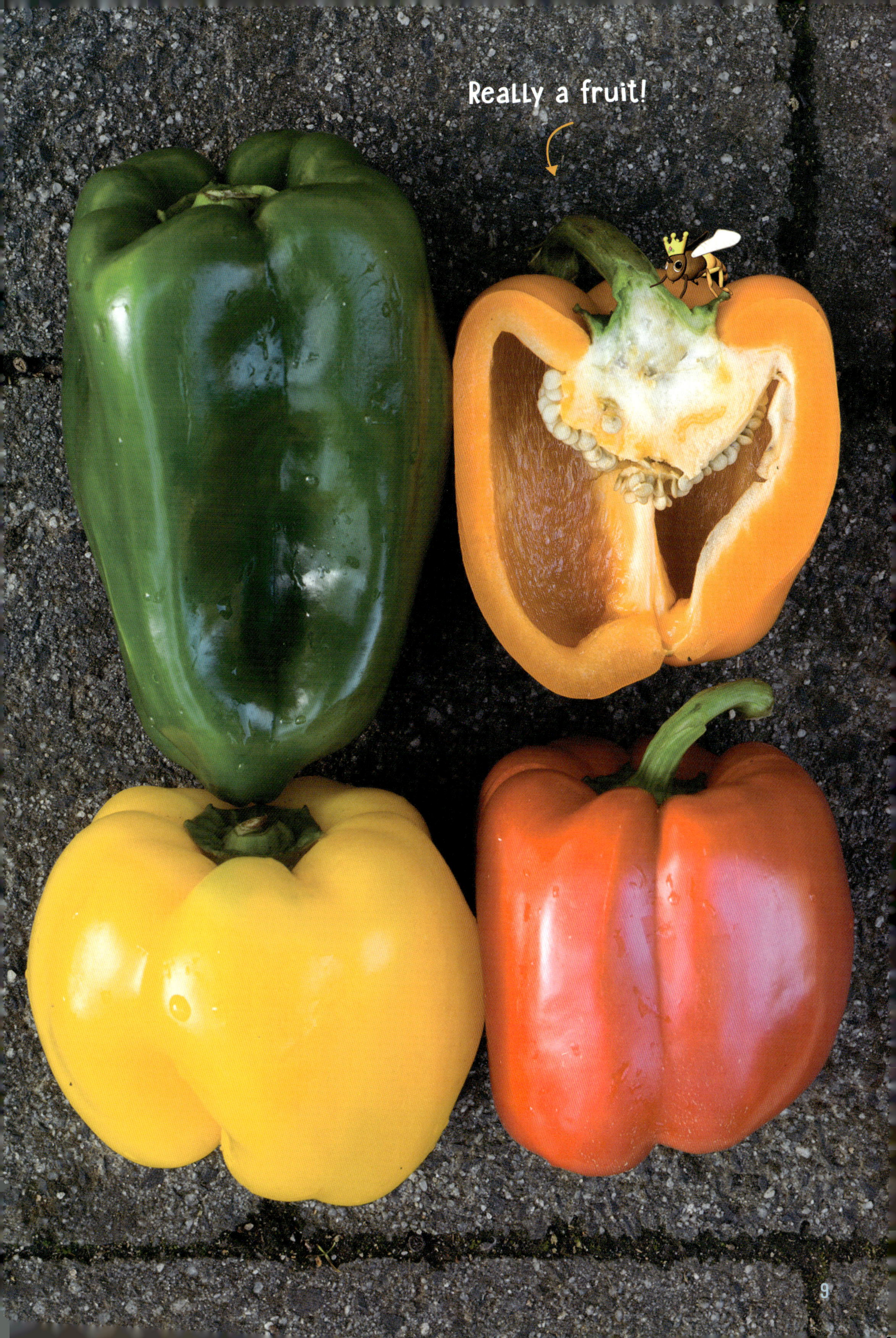
Really a fruit!

BEANS

In Season

Summer

and

Autumn

Grows How?

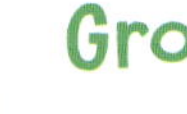

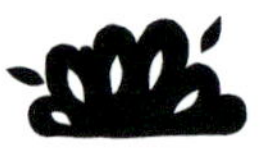

In bushes

A Serve

1/2 cup

Good For Your

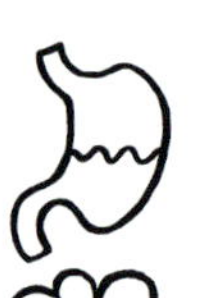

tummy

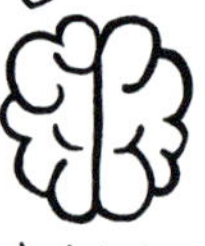

brain

heart

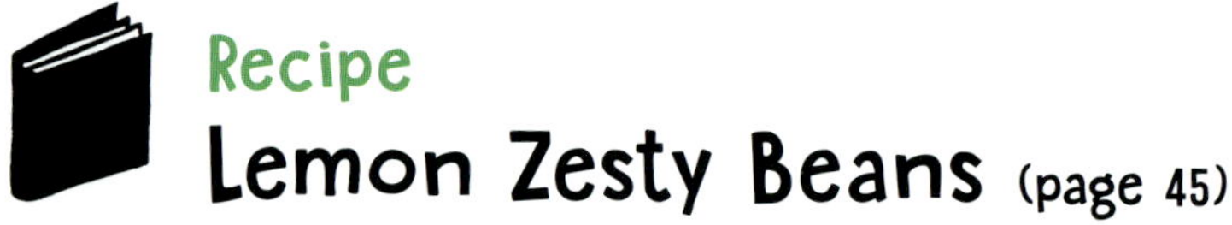

Recipe

Lemon Zesty Beans (page 45)

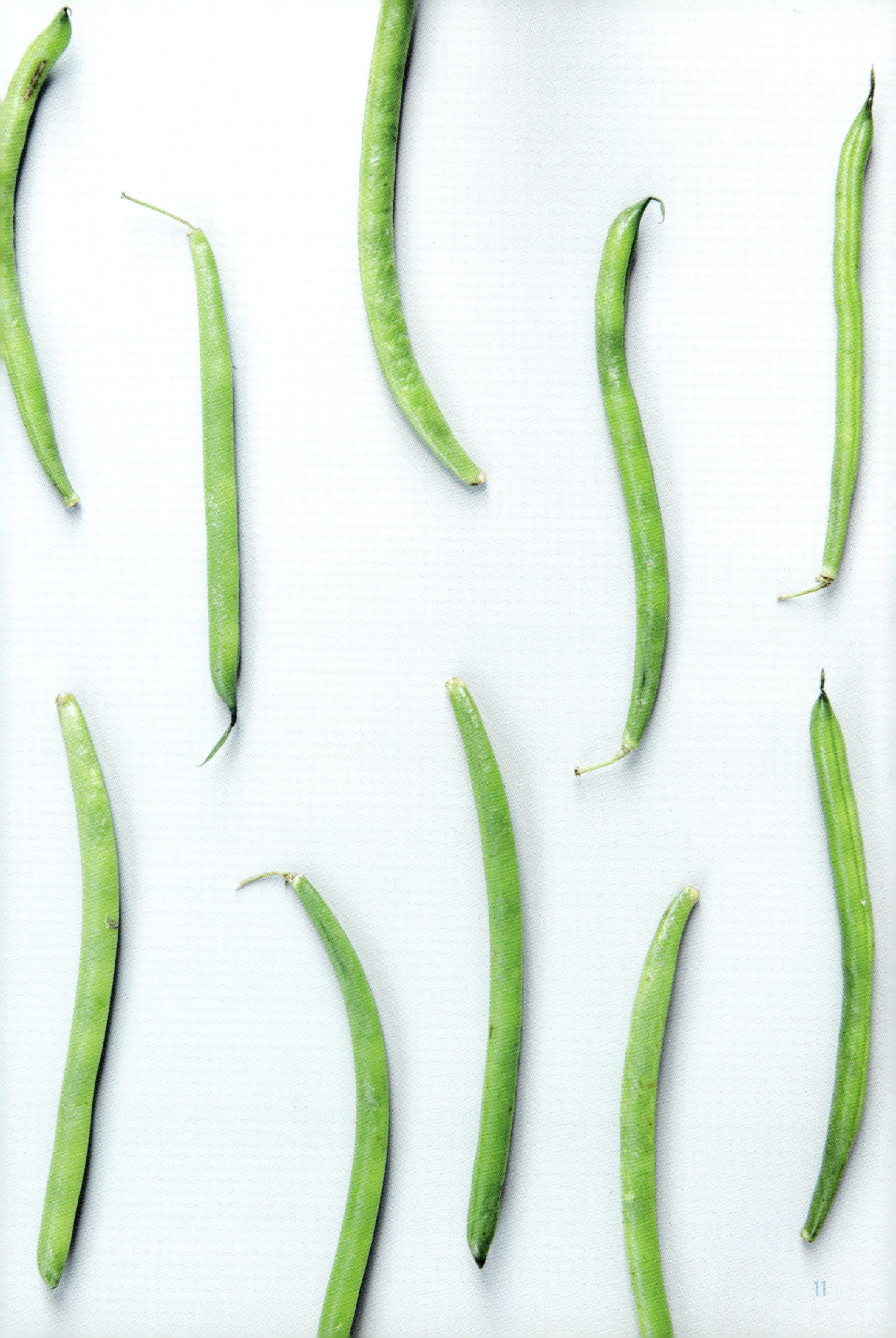

SNOW PEAS

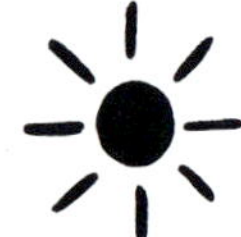

In Season

Summer

and

Autumn

Grows How?

On vines

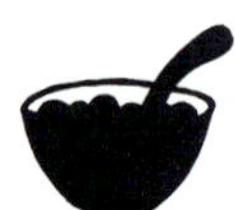

A Serve

1/2 cup

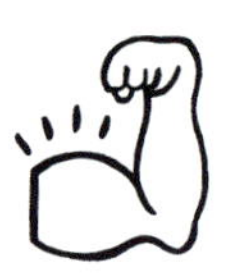

Good For Your

strength

heart

Recipe

Fresh Snow Peas (page 44)

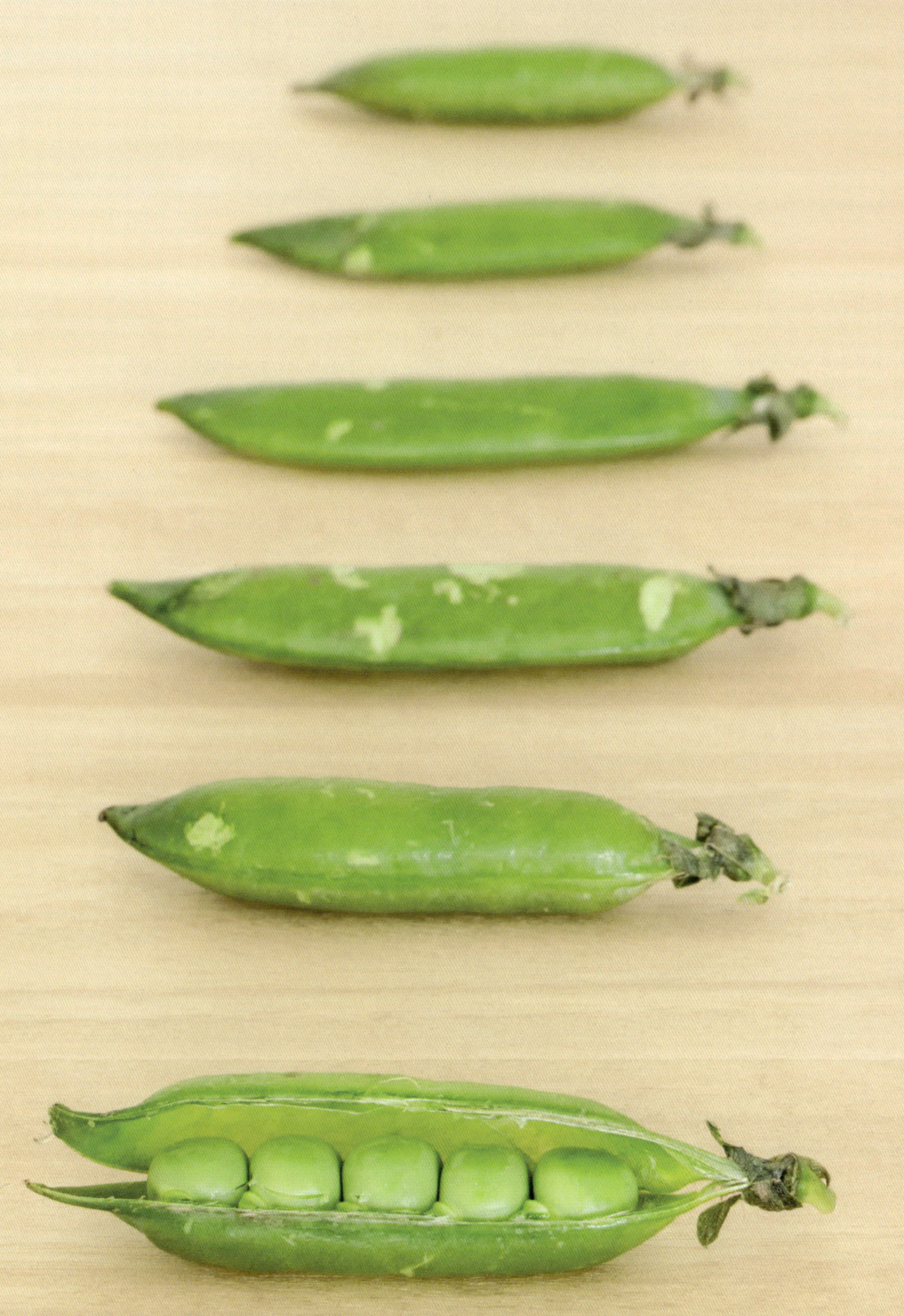

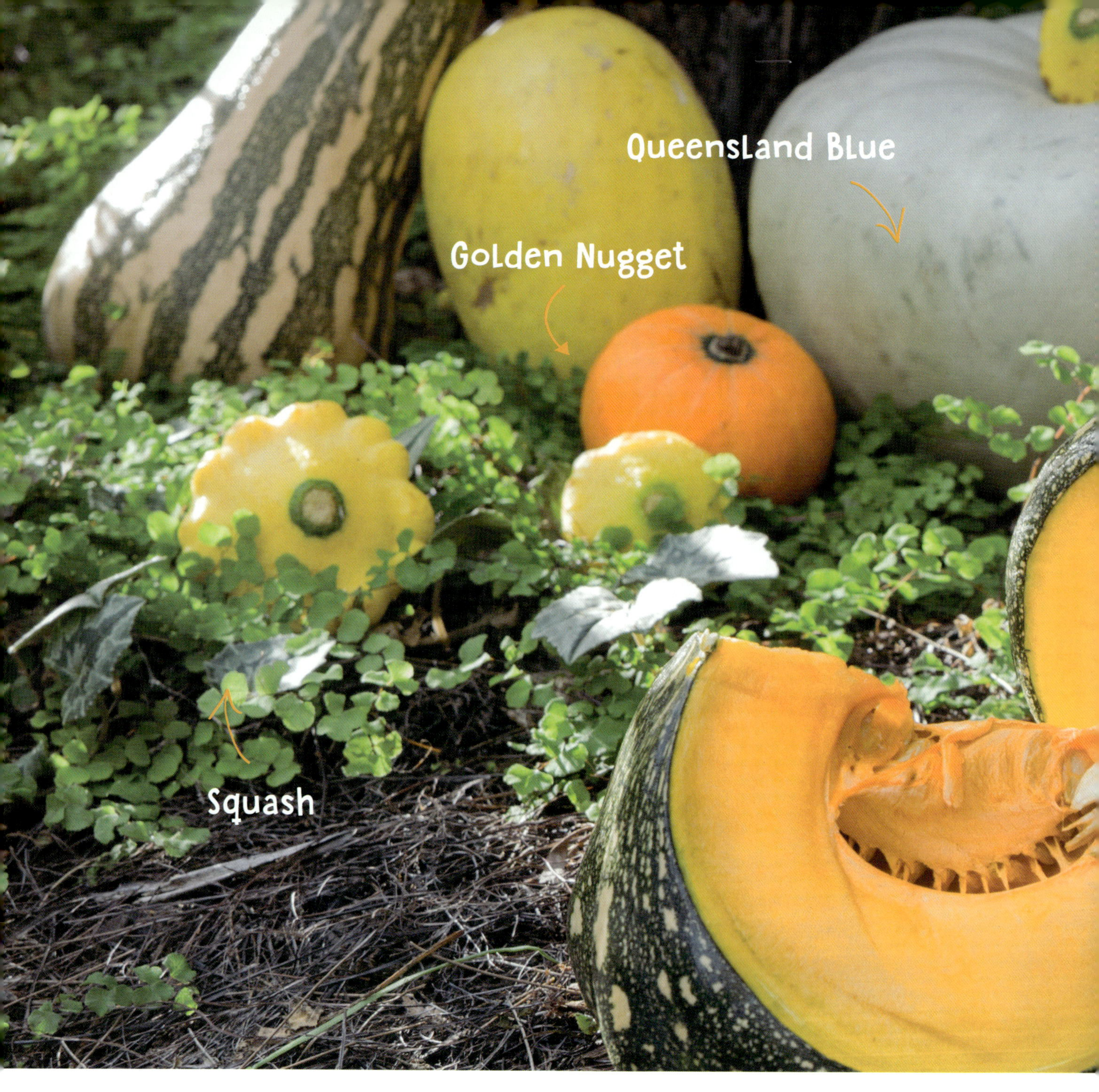

PUMPKIN

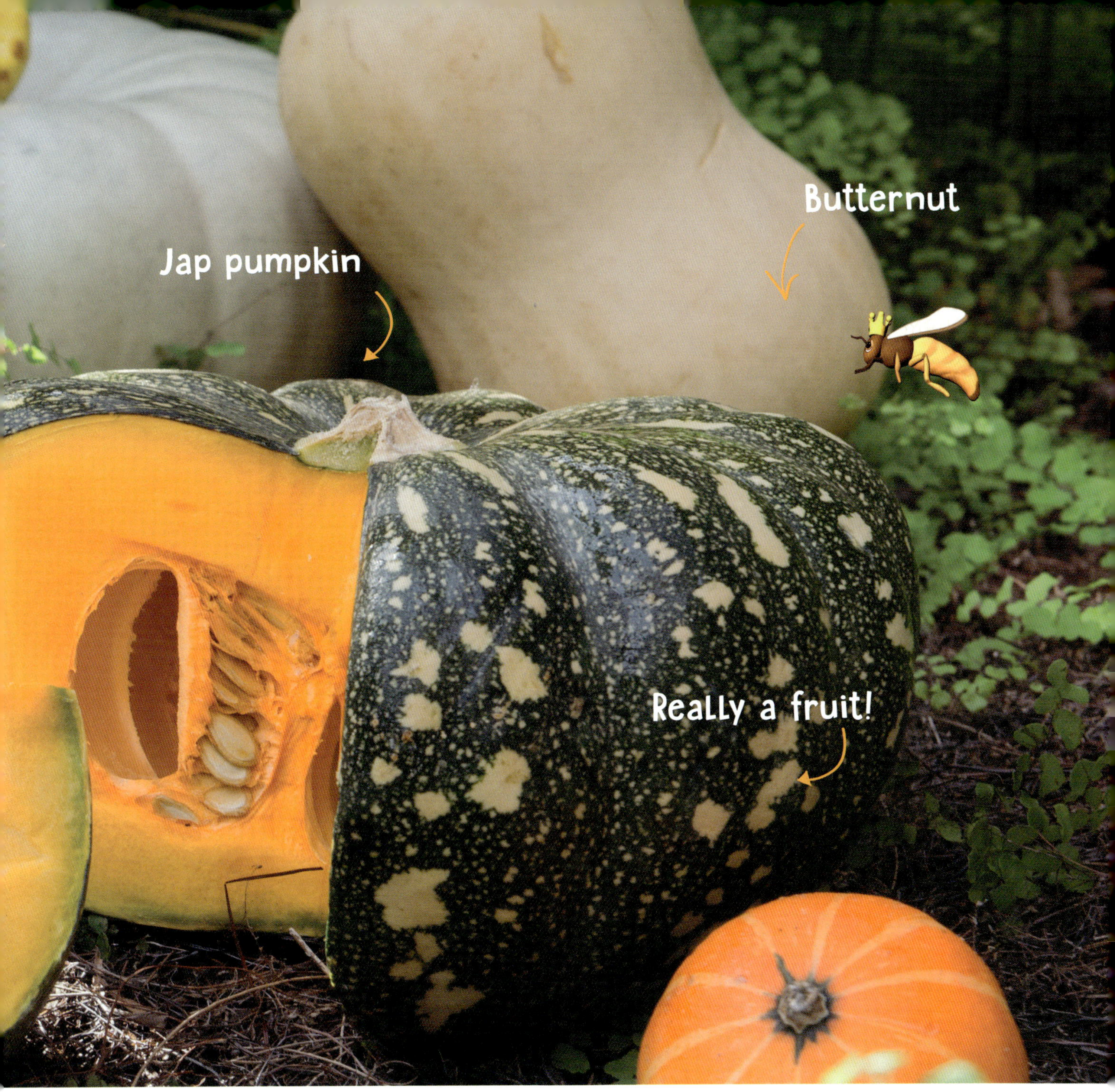

Butternut

Jap pumpkin

Really a fruit!

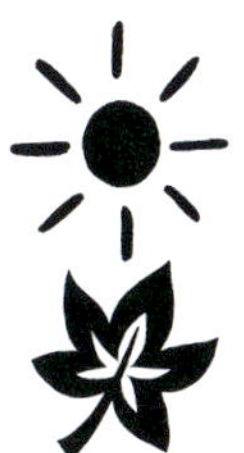

In Season

Summer

and Autumn

Grows How?

On vines

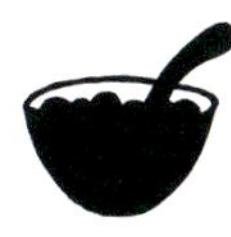

A Serve

1/2 cup

Good For Your

eyes

heart

strength

energy

Recipe

Amazing Pumpkin Soup

(page 49)

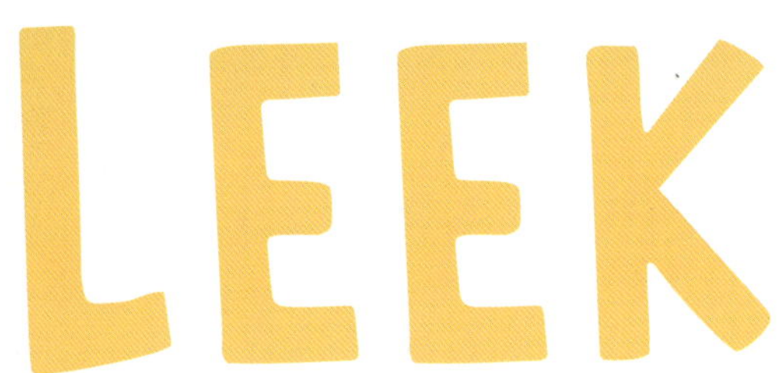

LEEK

In Season

Summer

and

Spring

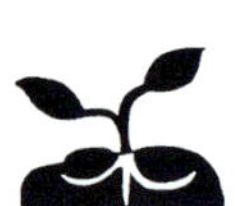

Grows How?

In the ground

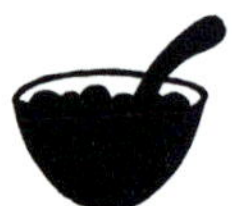

A Serve

1/2 cup

Good For Your

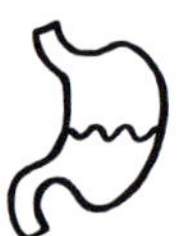

tummy

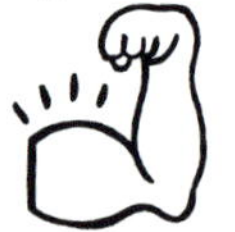

strength

heart

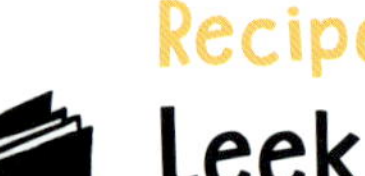

Recipe

Leek and Chick Pea Fritters with Tzatziki (page 46)

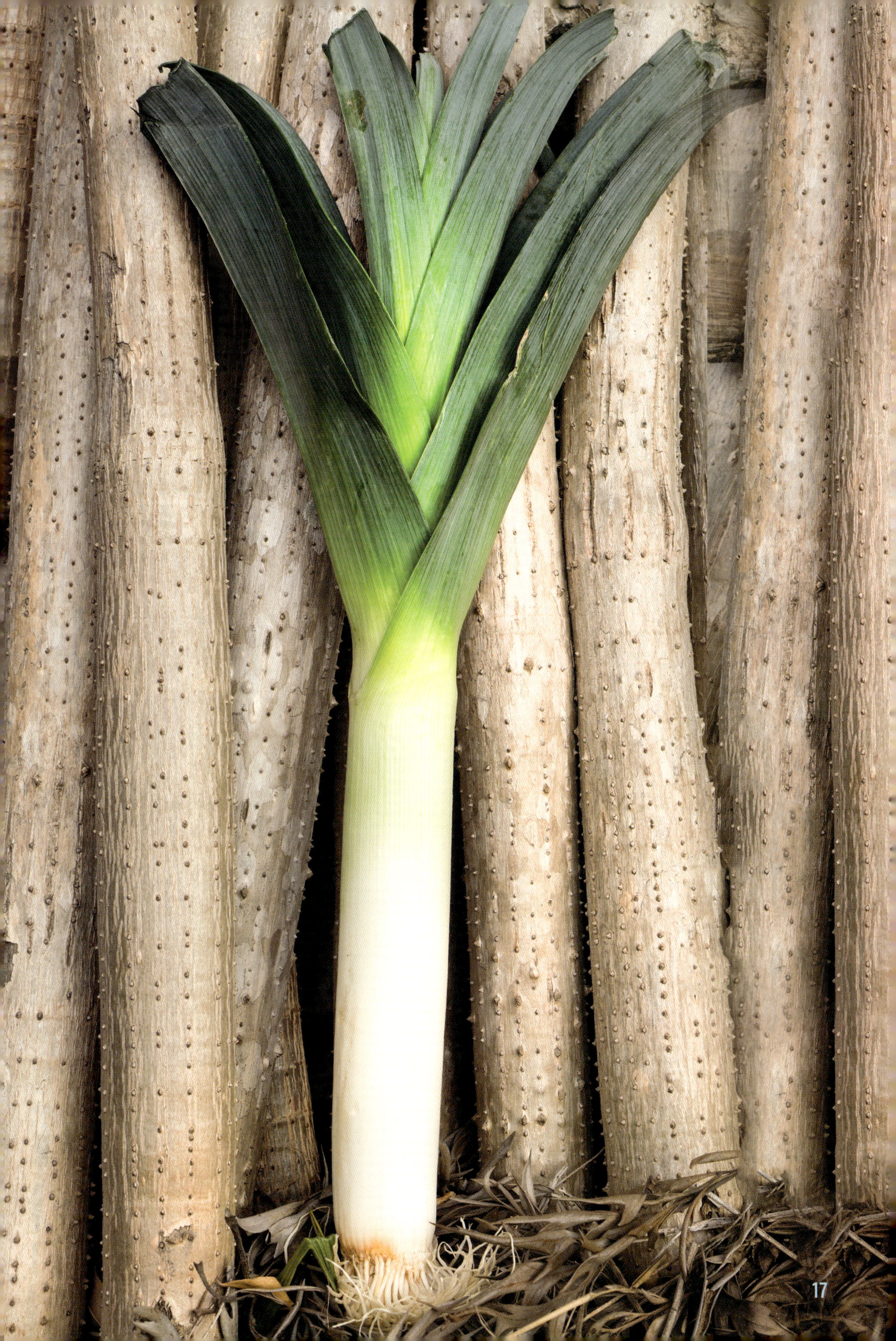

RHUBARB

In Season
Summer
and

Spring

Grows How?
In the ground

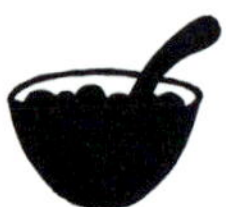

A Serve
1 cup

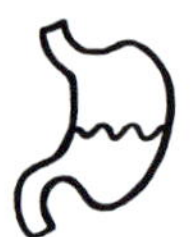

Good For Your
tummy

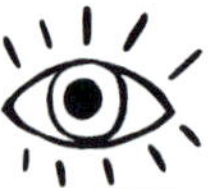

eyes

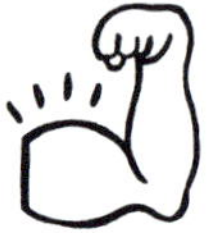

strength

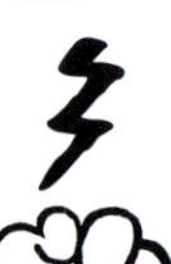

energy

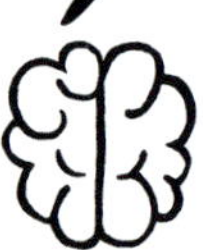

brain

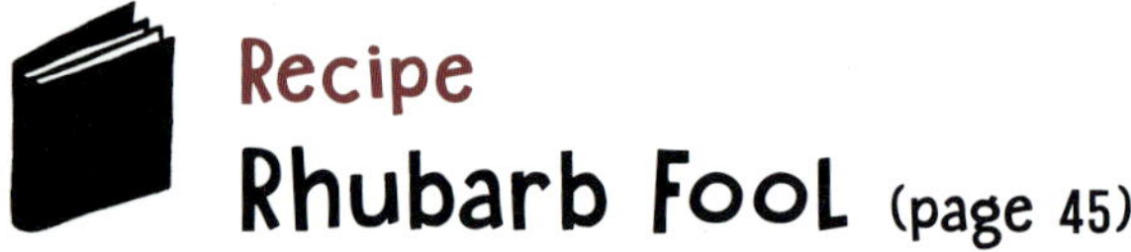

Recipe
Rhubarb Fool (page 45)

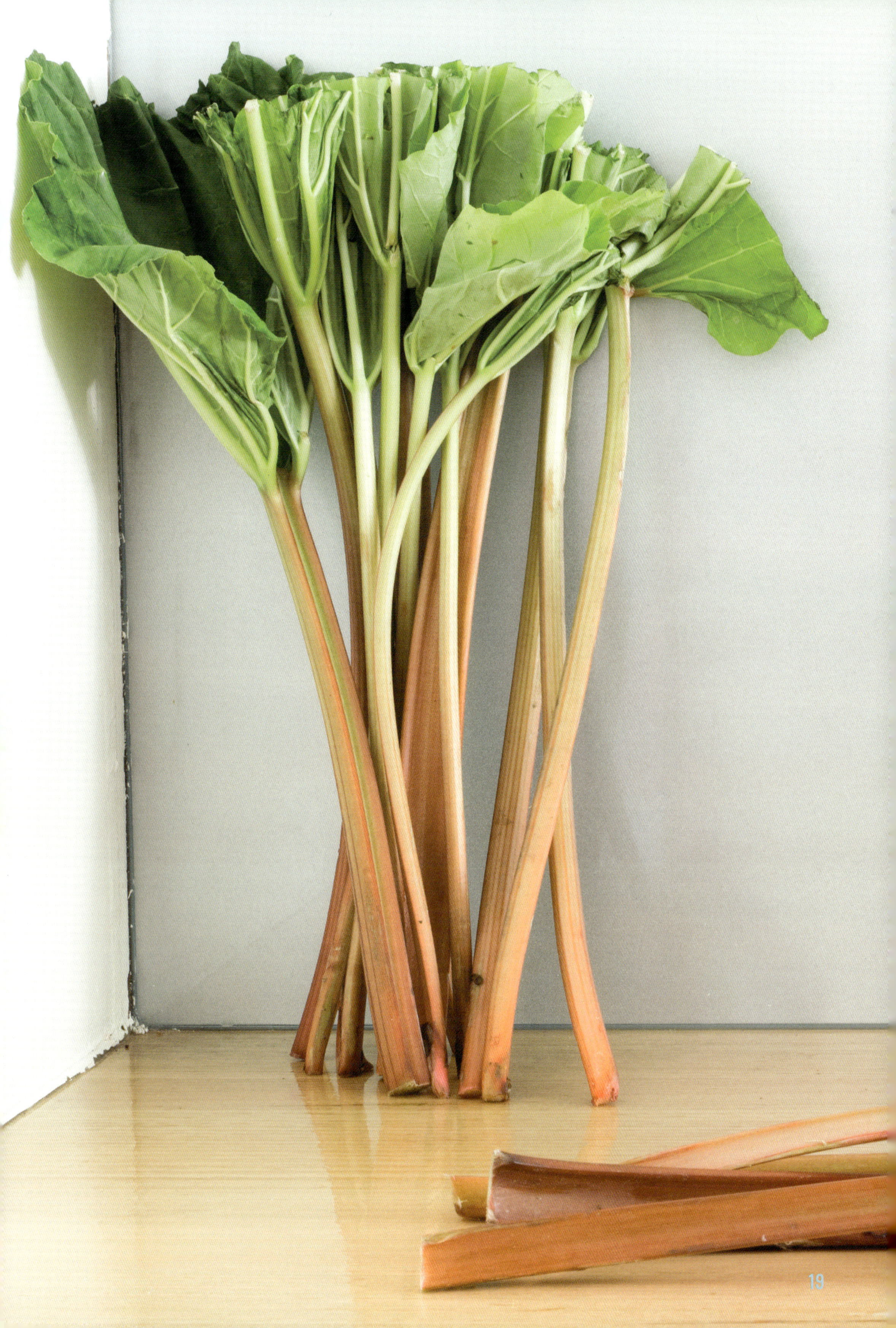

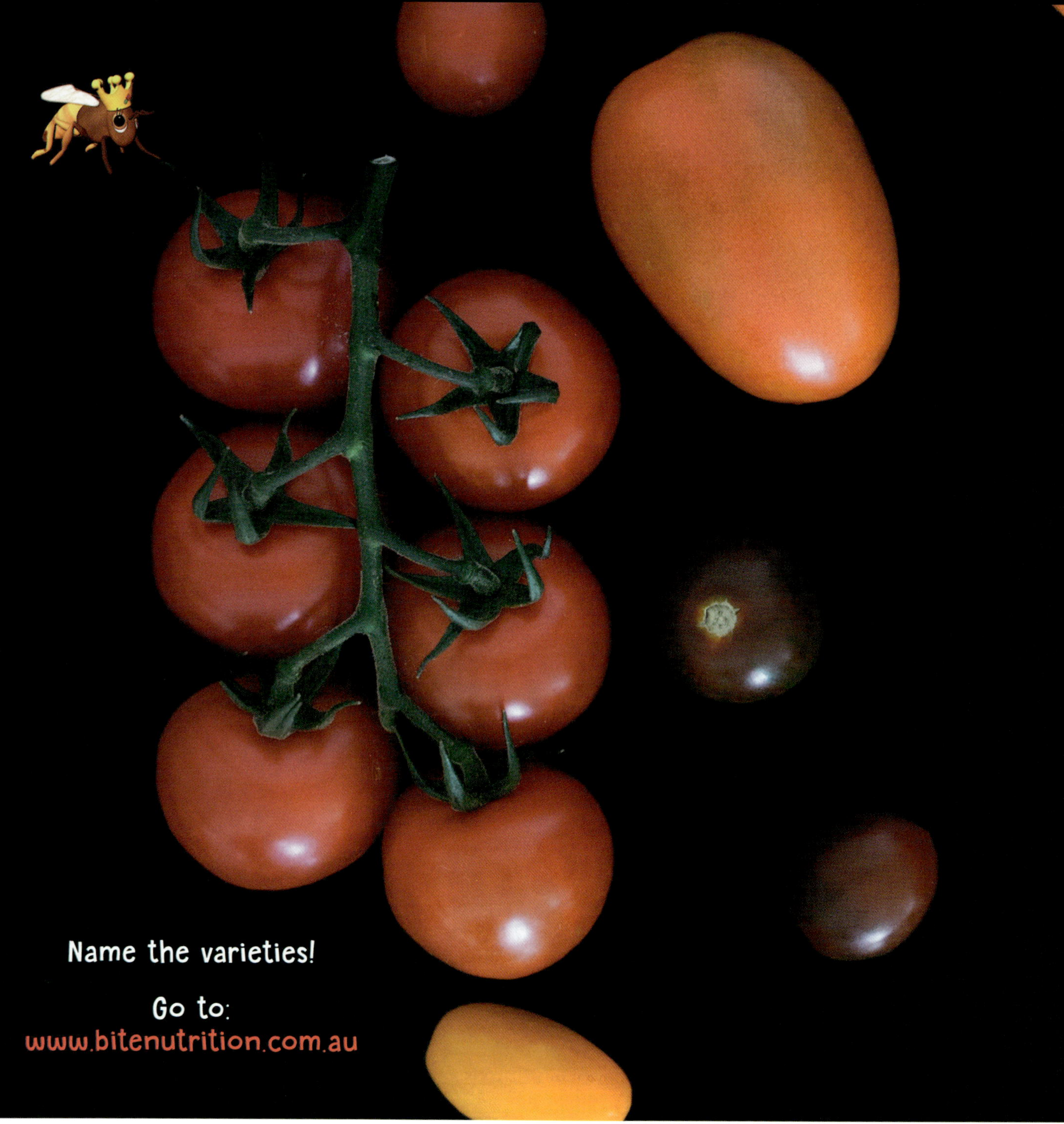

TOMATO

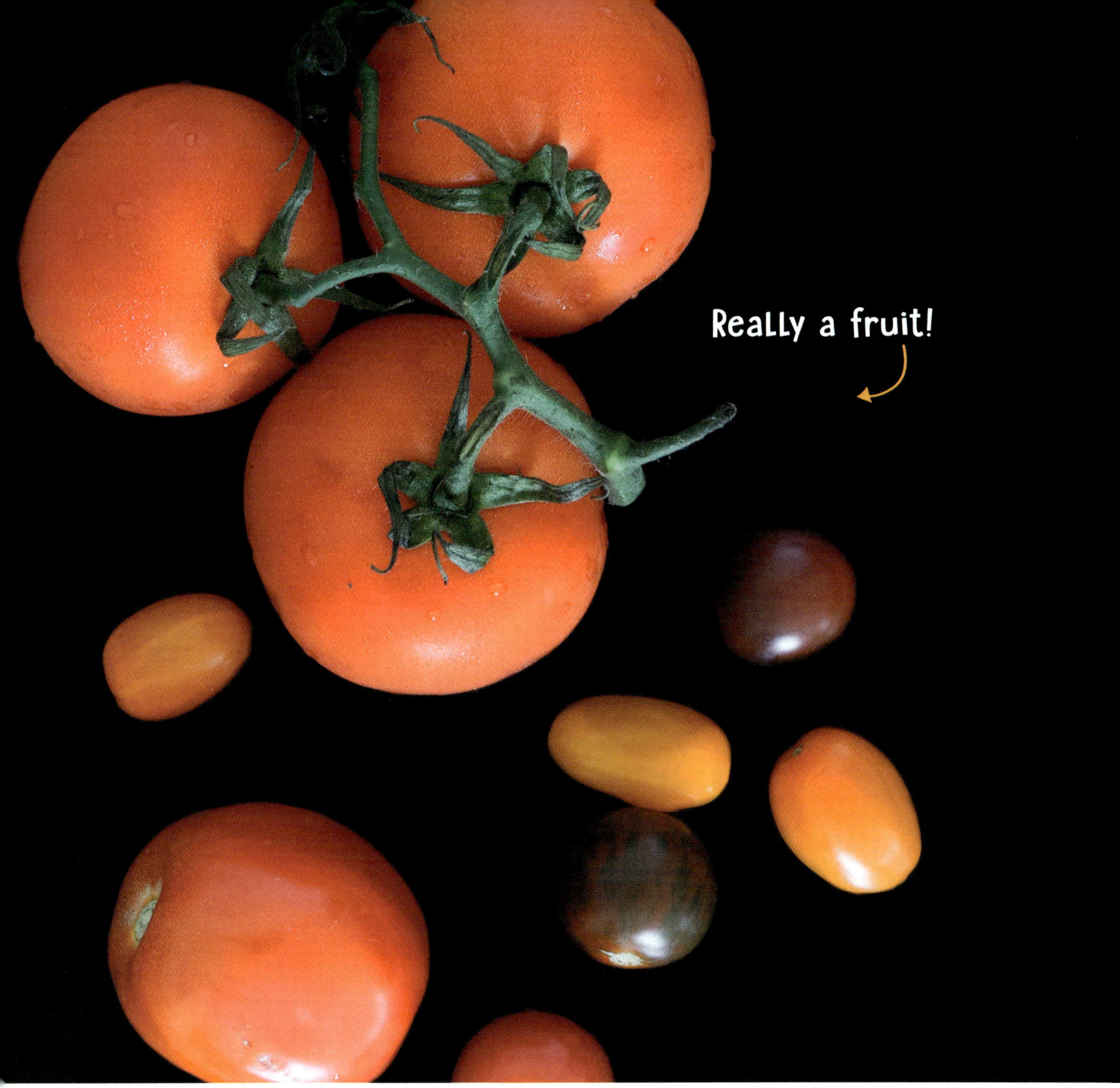

Really a fruit!

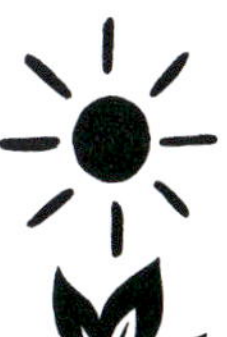

In Season

Summer

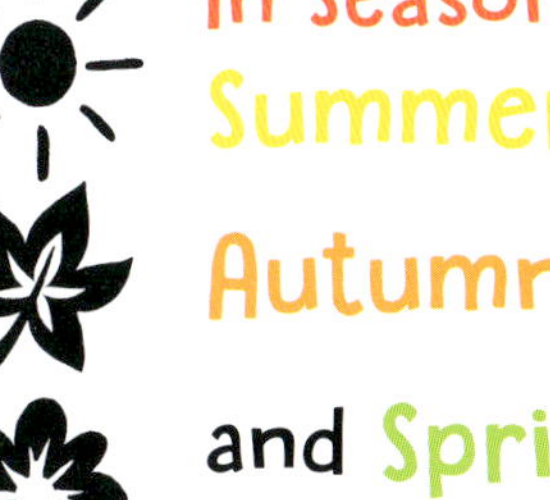

Autumn

and Spring

Grows How?

On vines

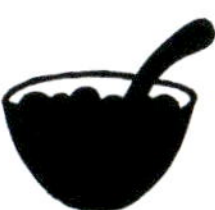

A Serve

1 cup

Good For Your

heart

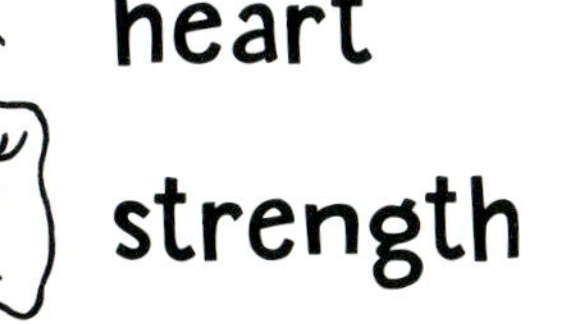

strength

brain

Recipe

Roasted Tomato Tart

(page 47)

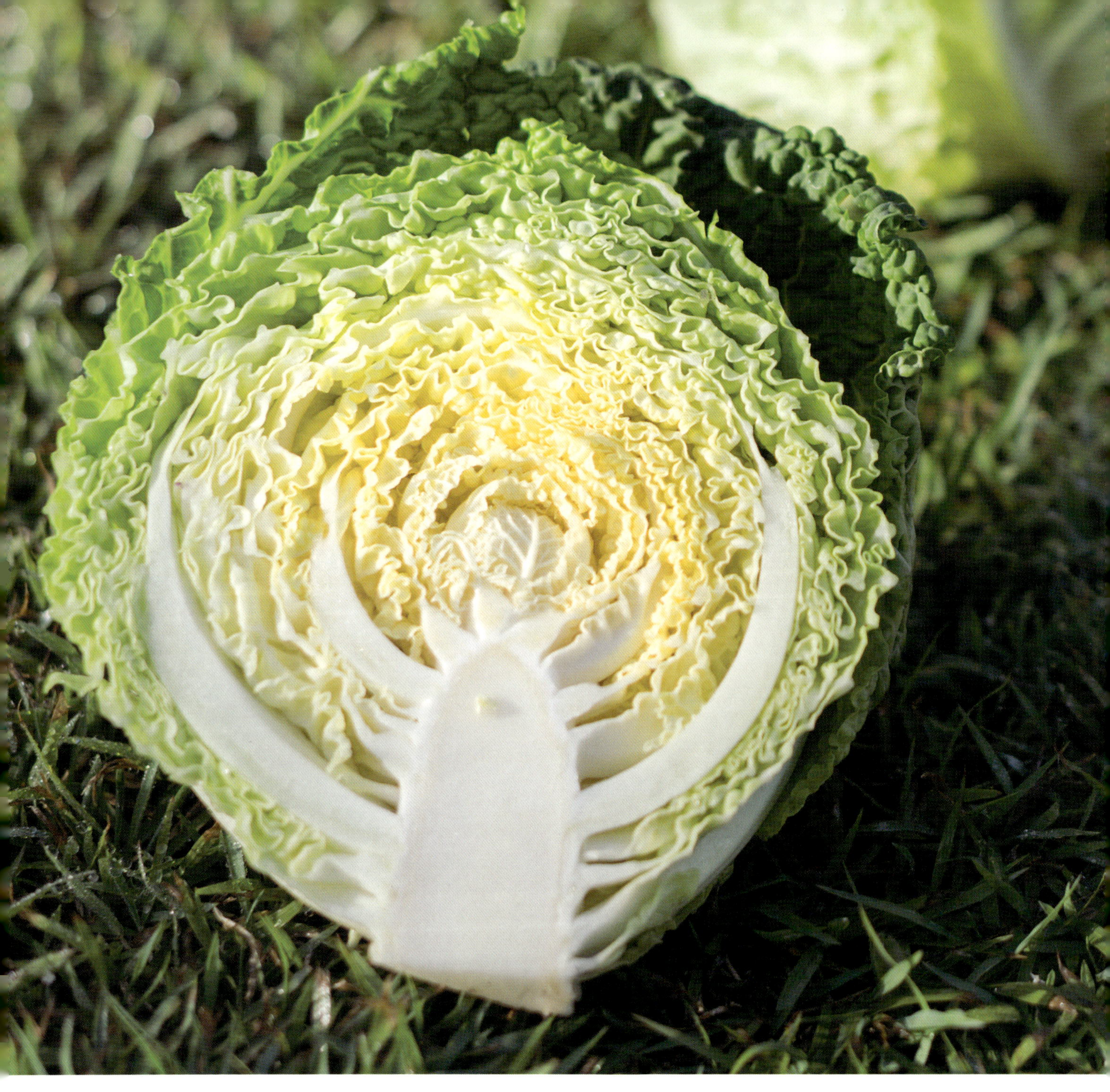

CABBAGE

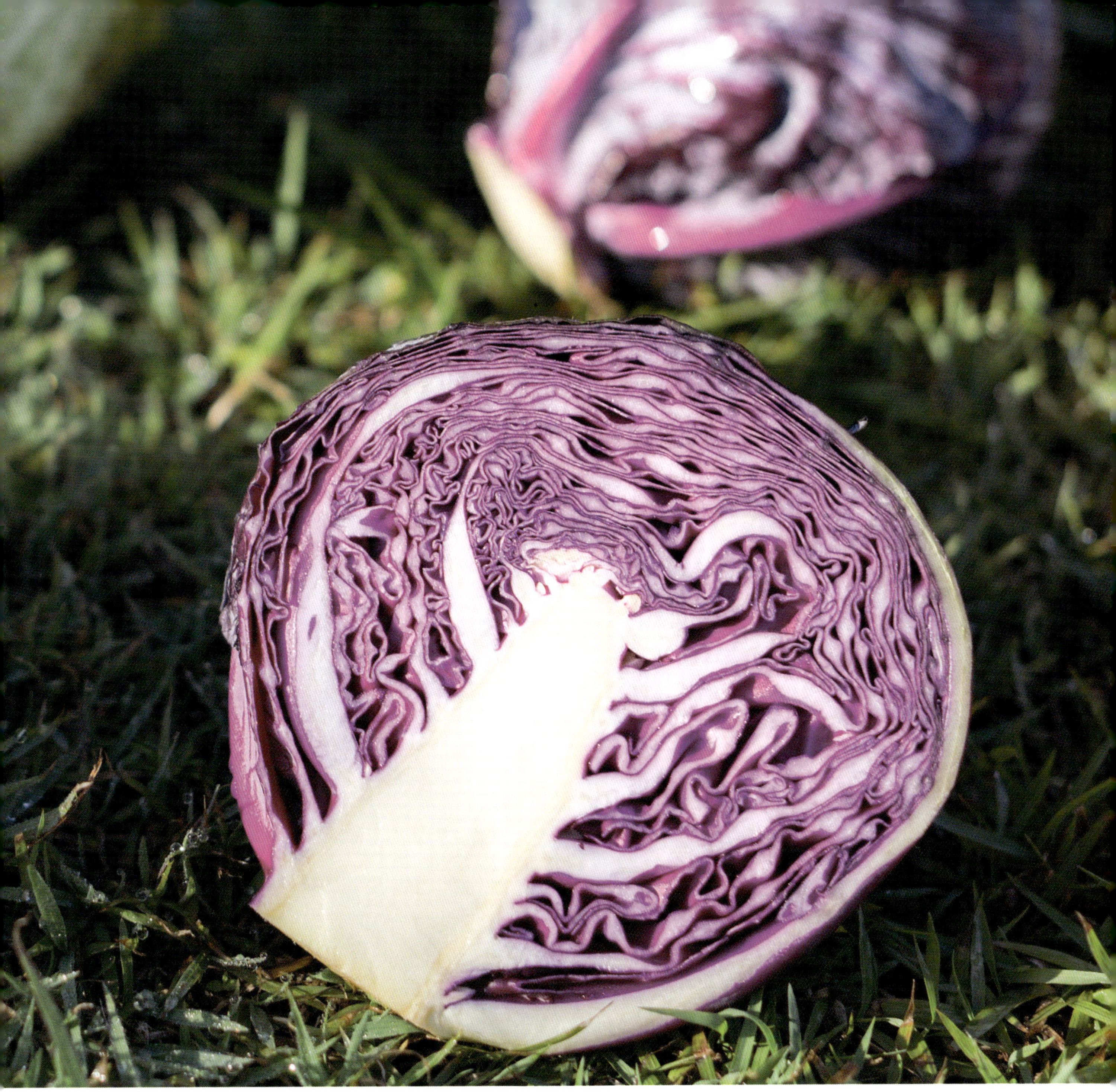

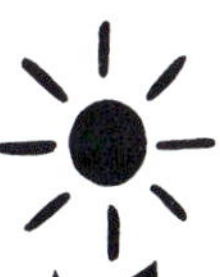
In Season
Summer

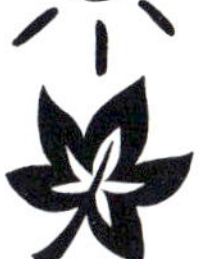
Autumn

and Spring

Grows How?

In the ground

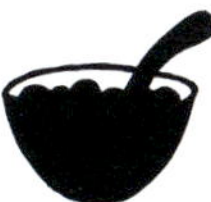
A Serve
1/2 cup

Good For Your

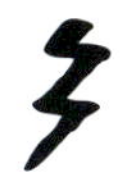
energy

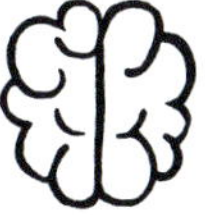
brain

Recipe

Cabbage Rolls (page 48)

BEETROOT

In Season

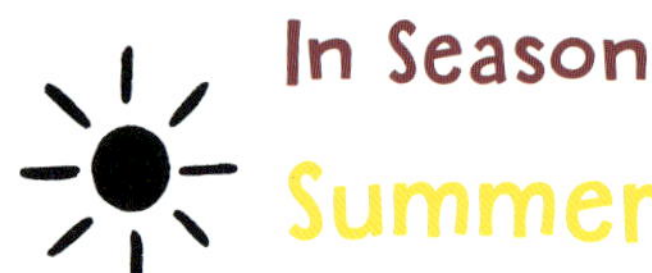 Summer, 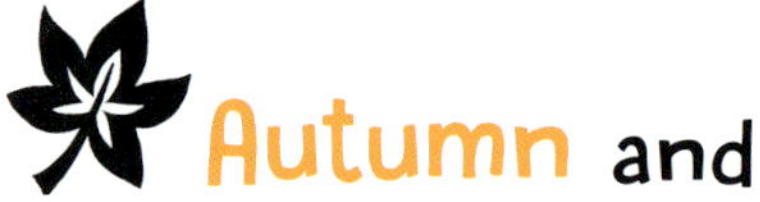 Autumn and 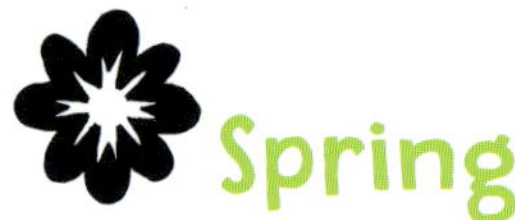 Spring

Grows How?

 In the ground

A Serve

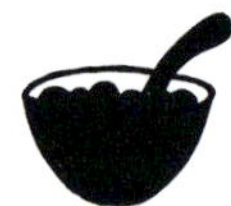 1/2 cup

Good For Your

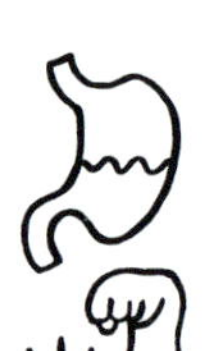 tummy

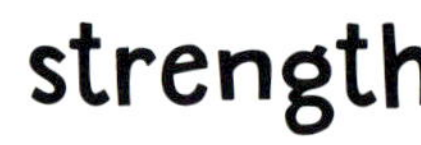

strength

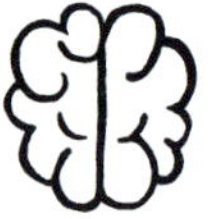 brain

Recipe

Beetroot Chips (page 43)

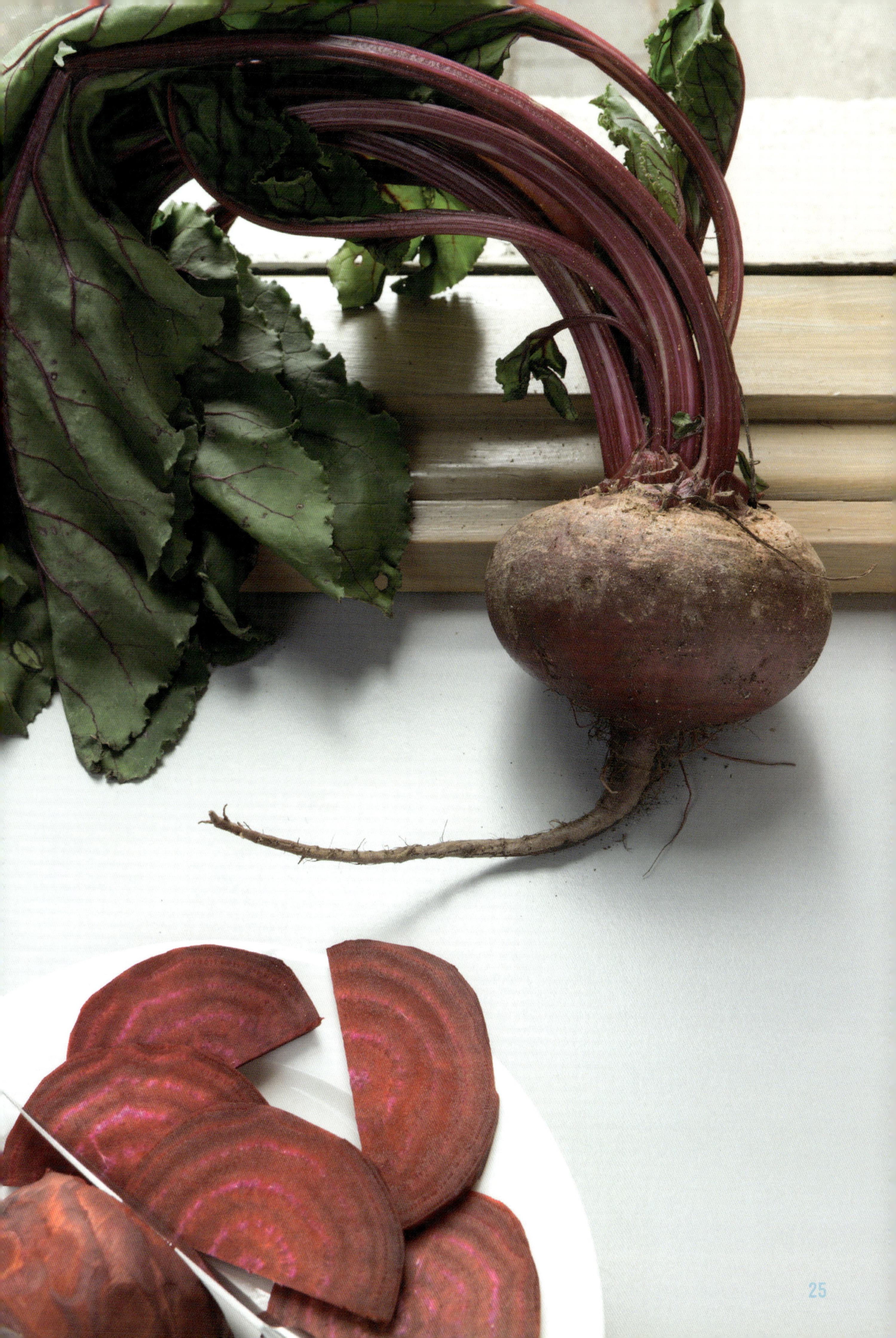

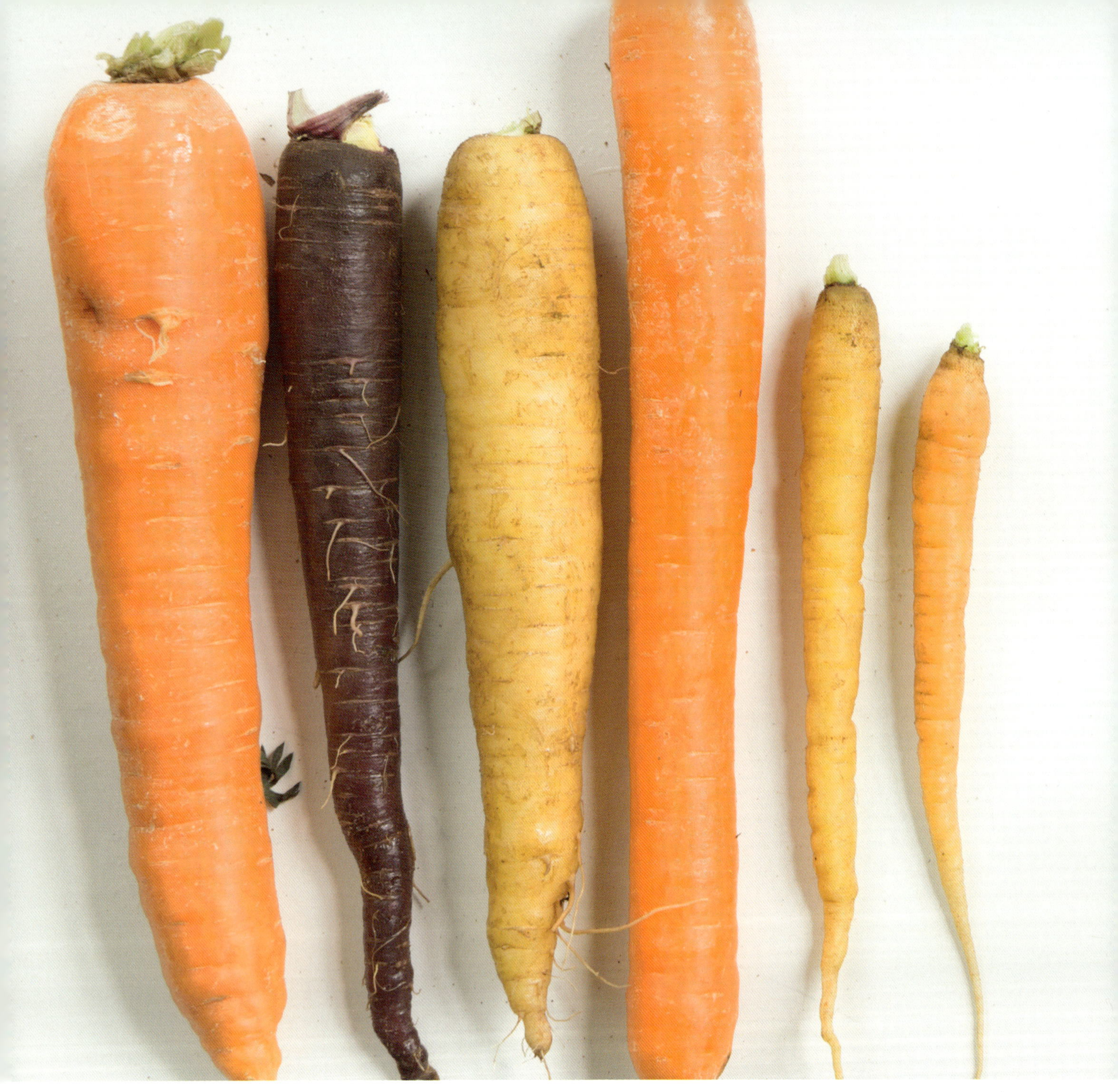

CARROT

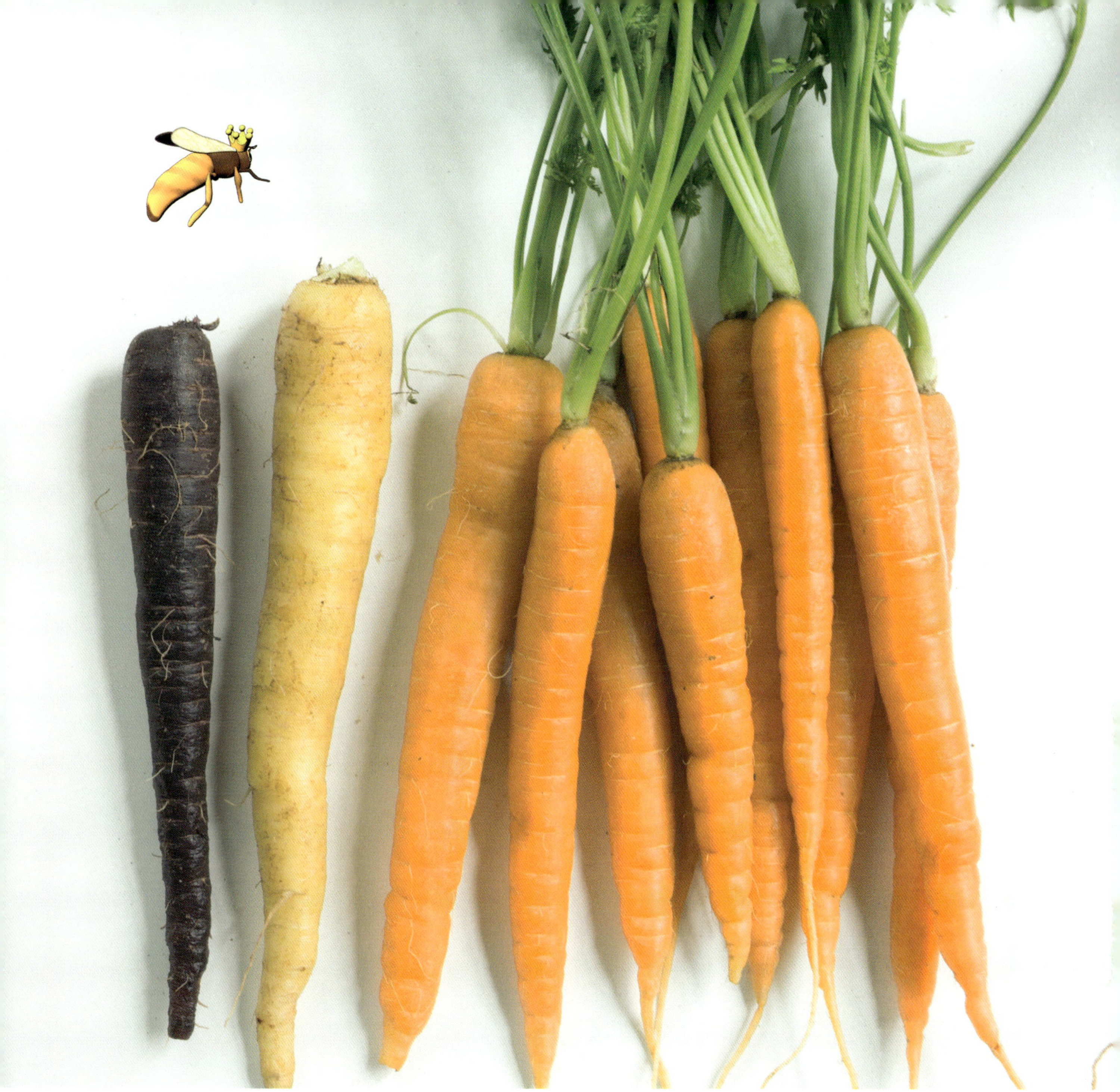

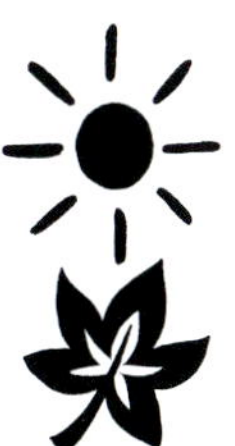

In Season
Summer
Autumn
and Winter

Grows How?

In the ground

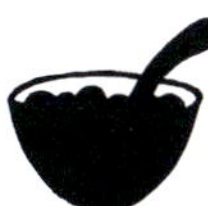

A Serve
1/2 cup

Good For Your

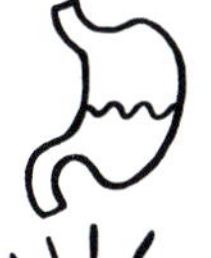

tummy
eyes

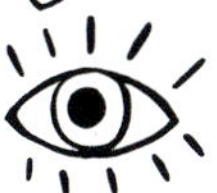

energy

heart

Recipe
Carrot Muffins
(page 43)

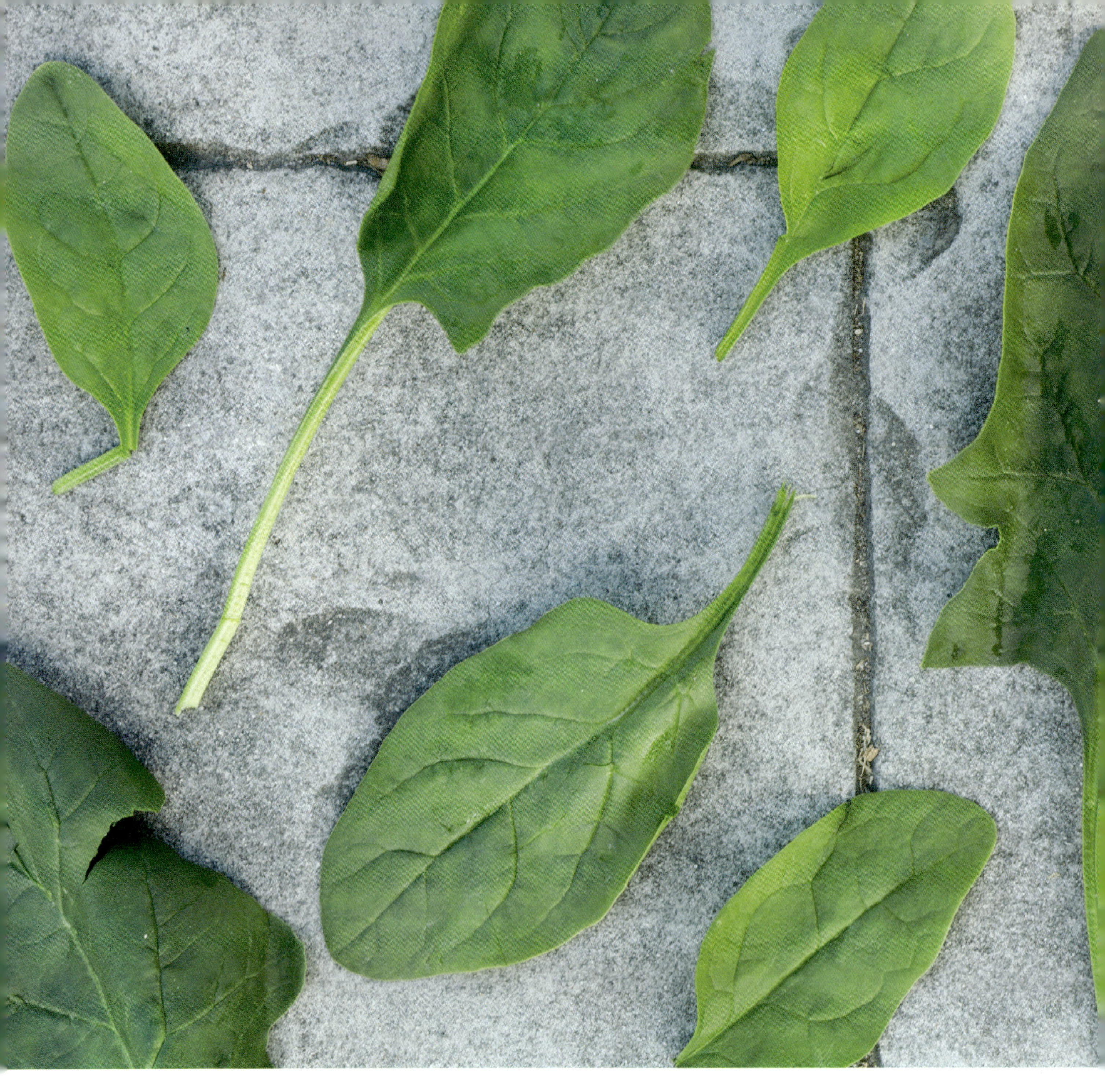

SPINACH

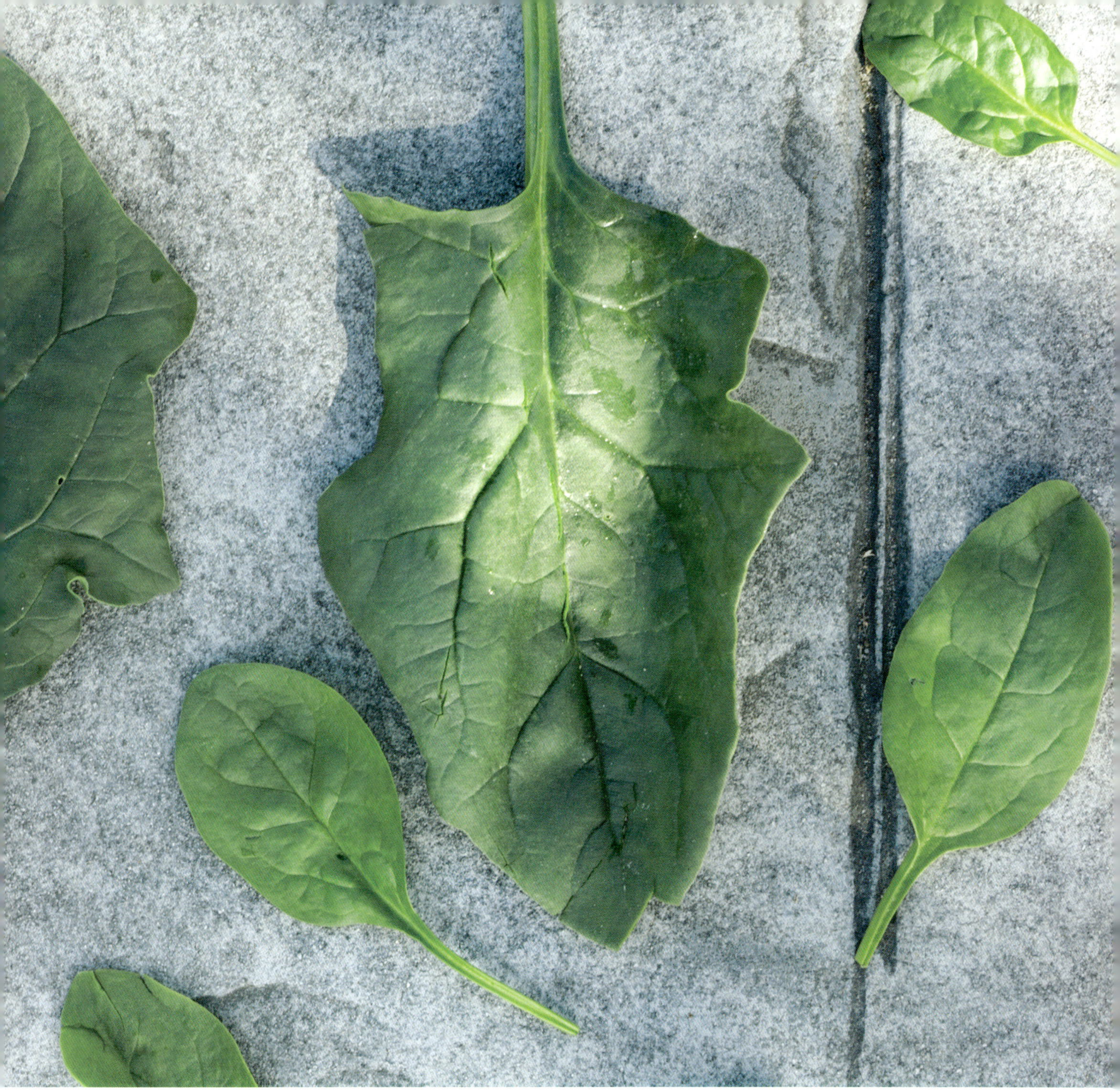

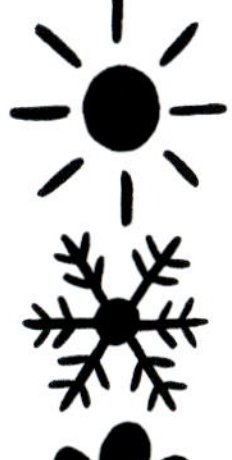

In Season
Summer
Winter
and Spring

Grows How?

In the ground

A Serve
1/2 cup

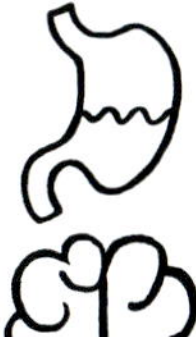

Good For Your
tummy

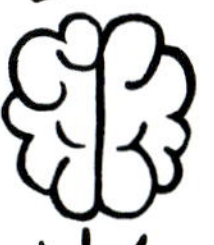

brain

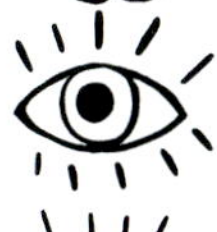

eyes

heart

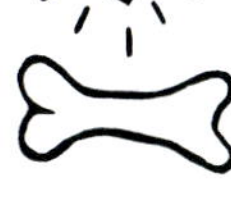

bones

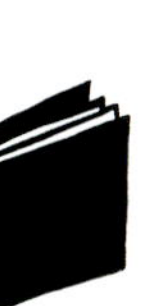

Recipe
Spinach and Ricotta Crepes
(page 44)

BRUSSEL SPROUTS

In Season

Winter

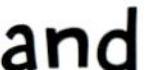
and

Spring

Grows How?

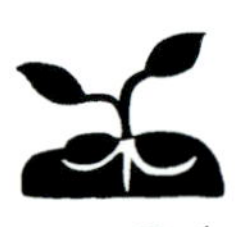
In the ground /
on a bush

A Serve

1/2 cup

Good For Your

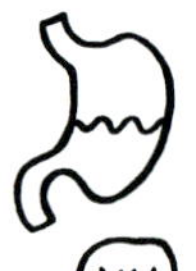
tummy

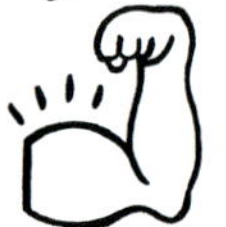
strength

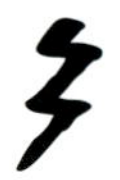
energy

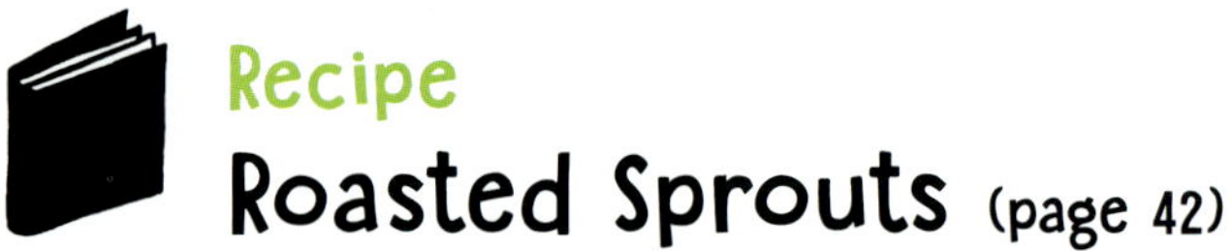
Recipe

Roasted Sprouts (page 42)

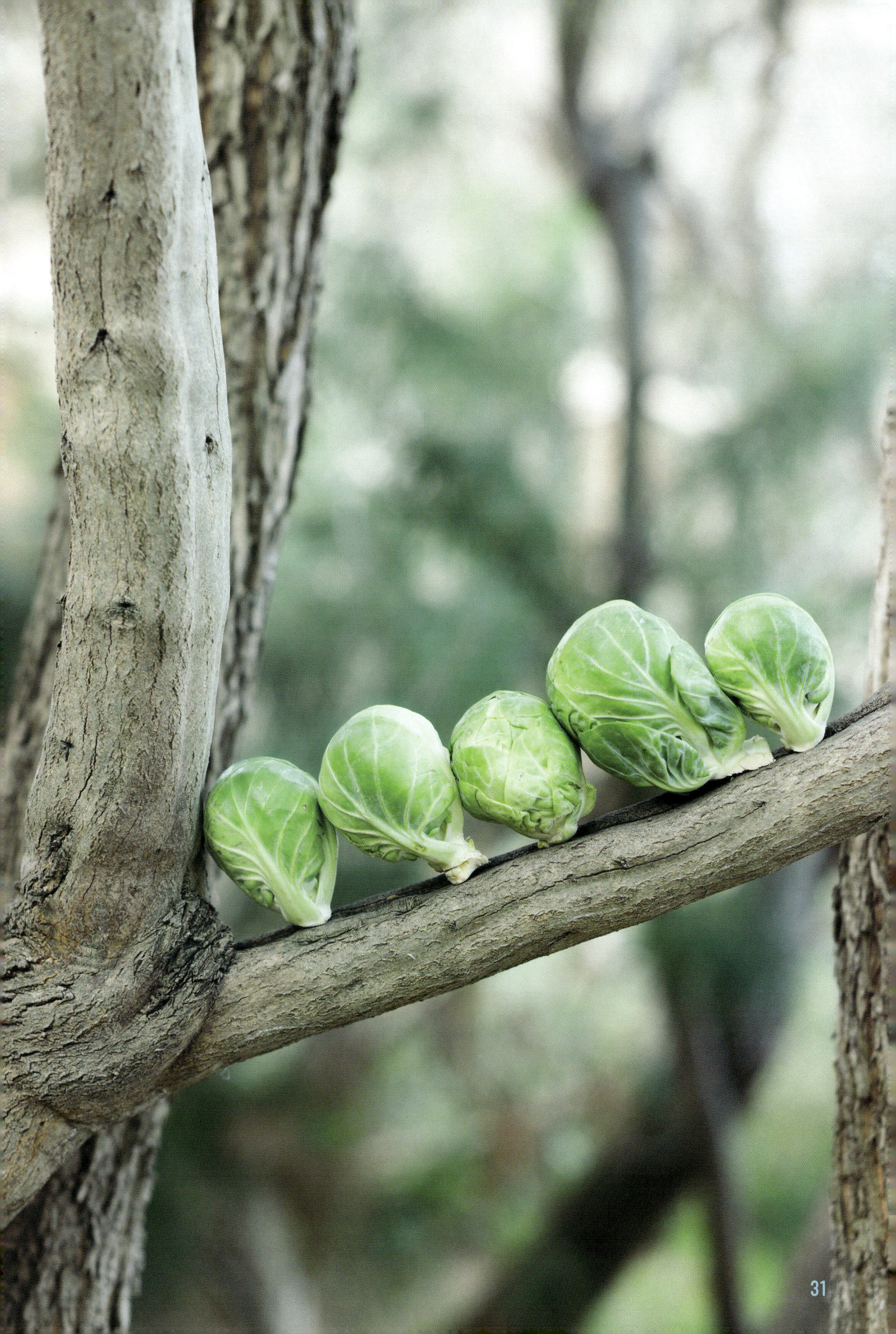

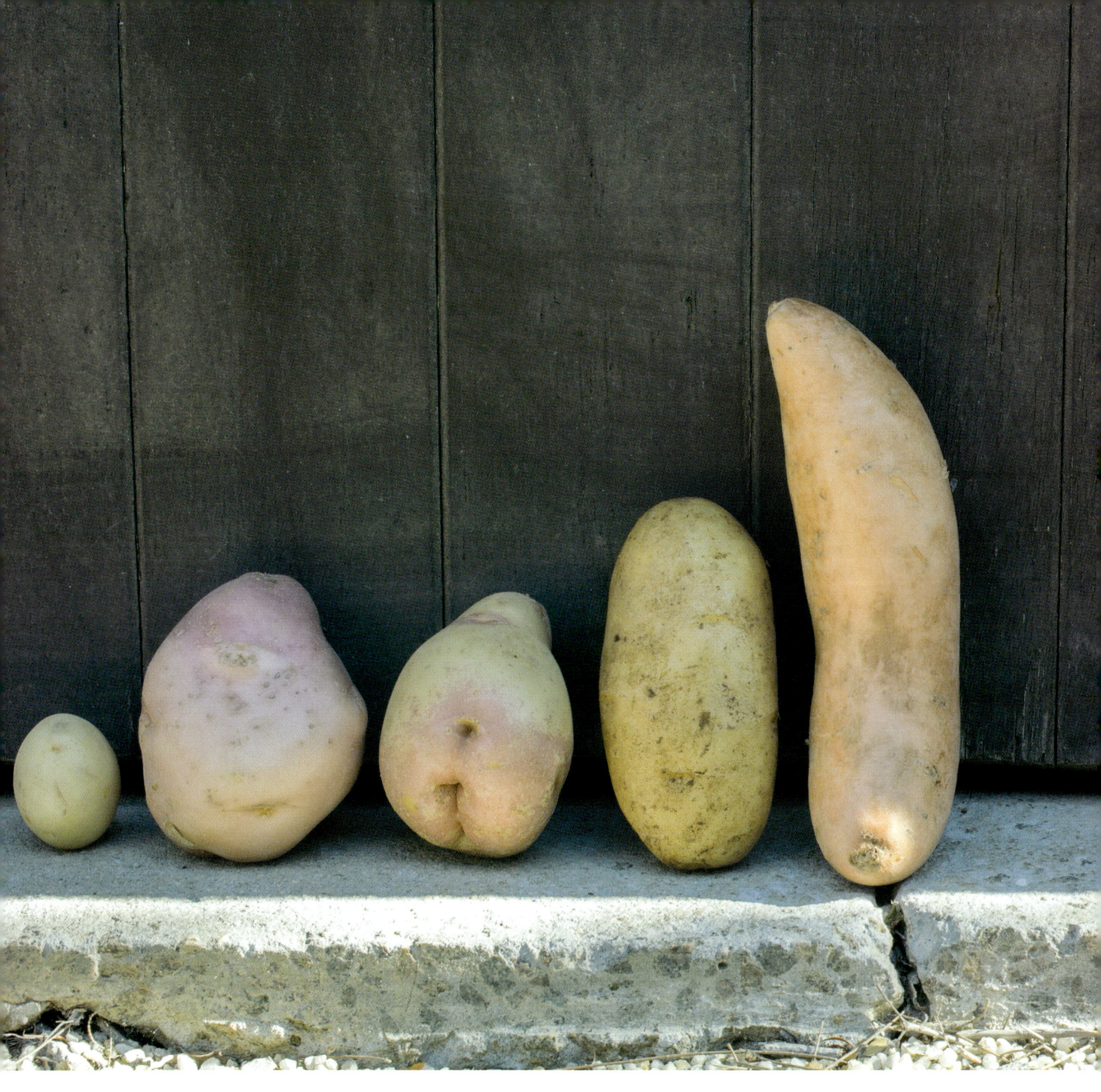

SWEET POTATO/ POTATO

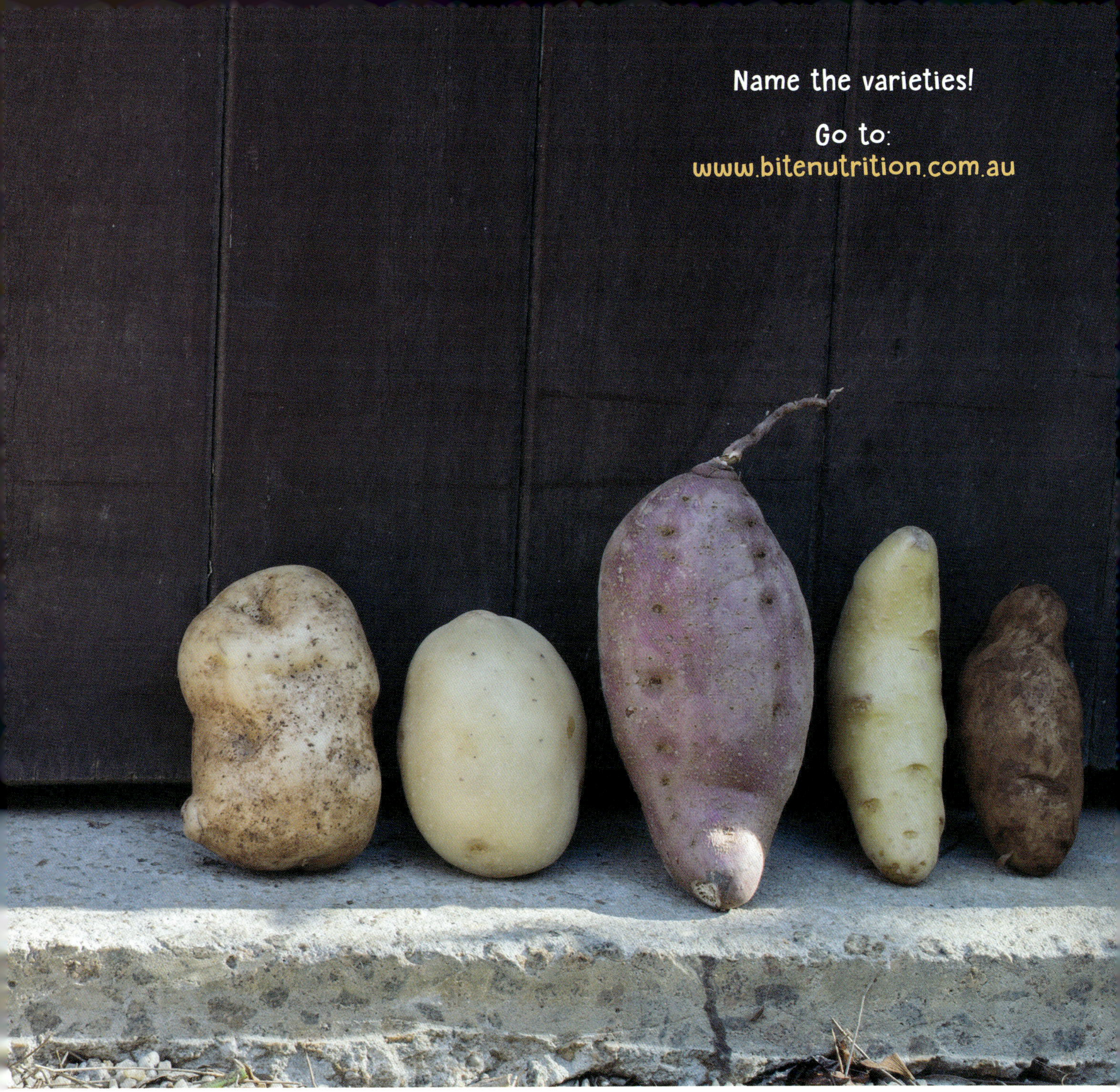

Name the varieties!

Go to:
www.bitenutrition.com.au

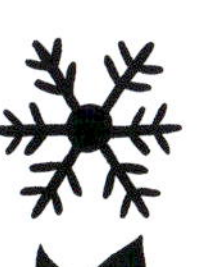
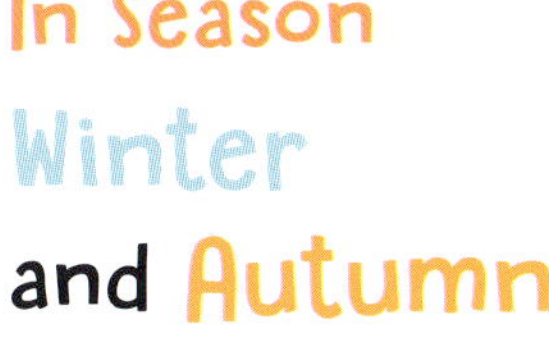

In Season

Winter and Autumn

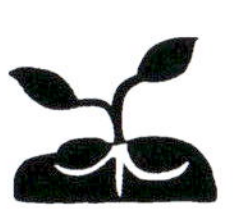

Grows How?

In the ground

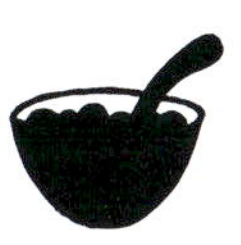

A Serve

½ cup

Good For Your (SWEET POTATO)

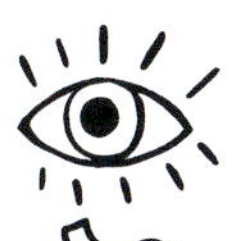
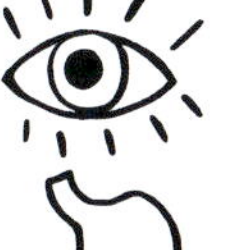

eyes

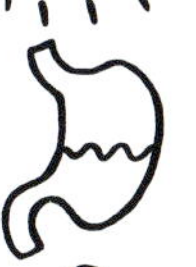

tummy

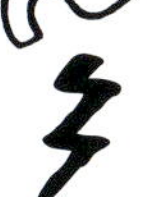

energy

Good For Your (POTATO)

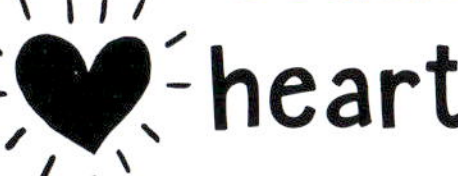

heart

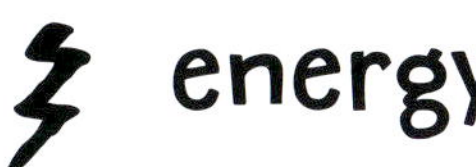

energy

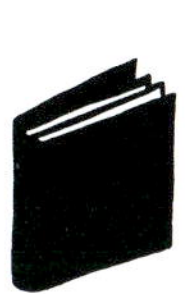

Recipe

Baked Potatoes

(page 52)

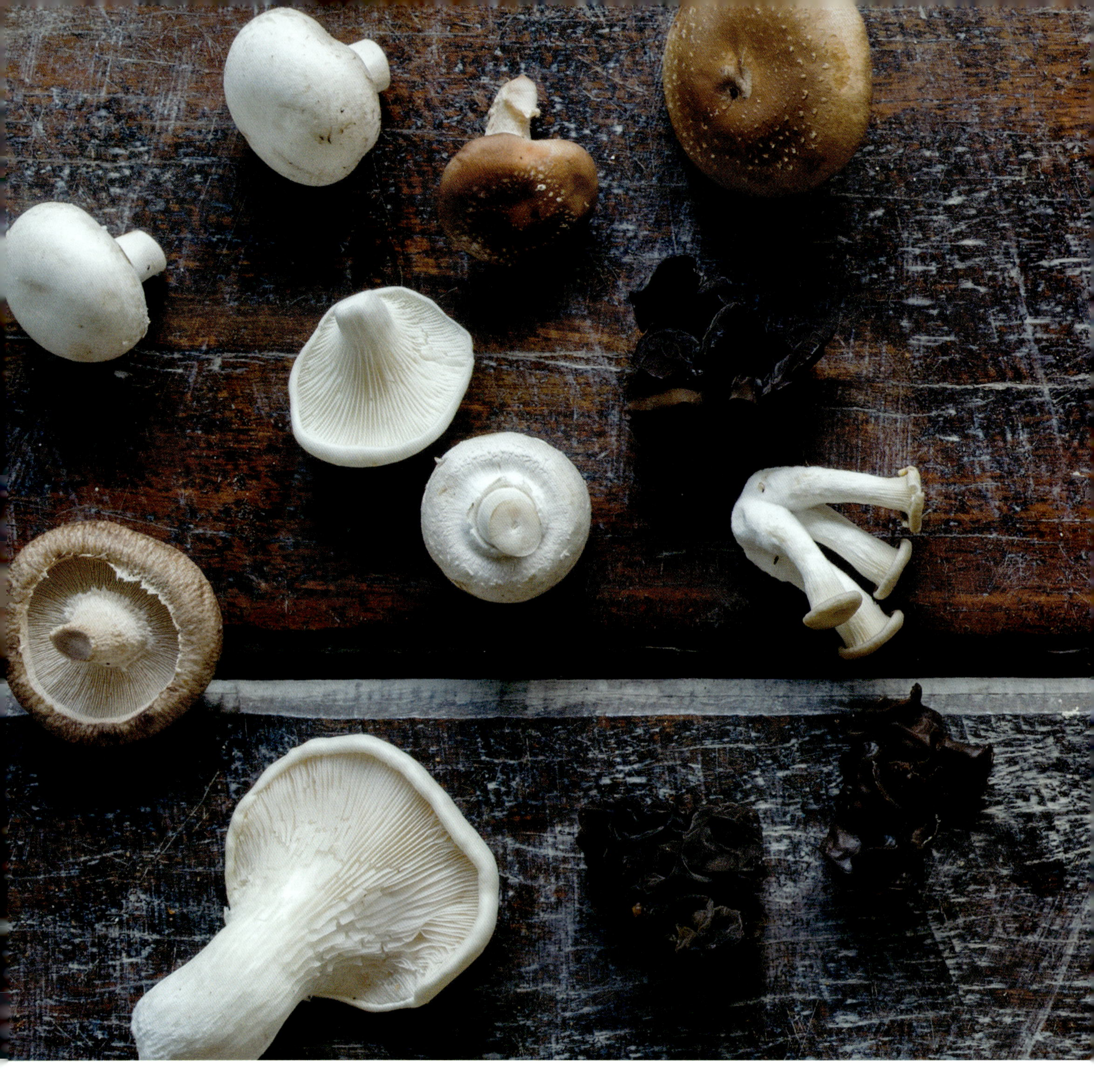

MUSHROOMS

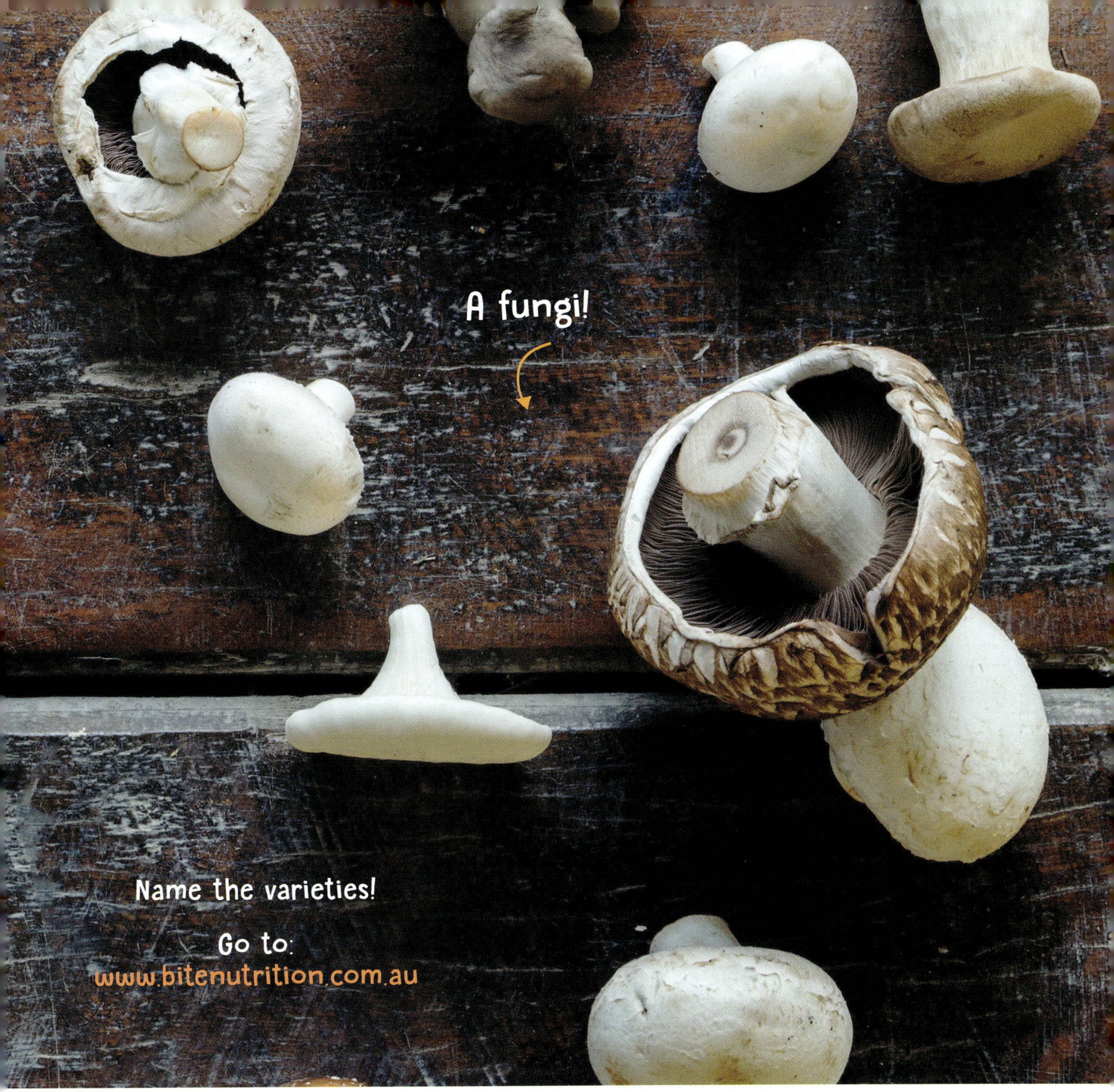

A fungi!

Name the varieties!

Go to:
www.bitenutrition.com.au

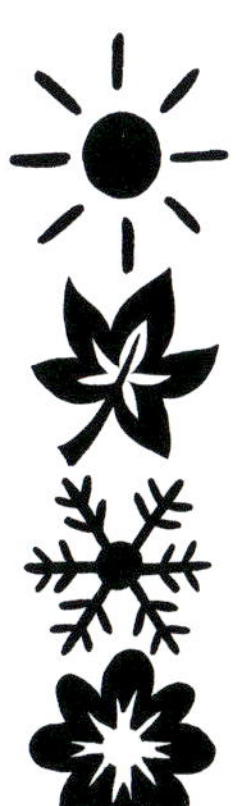

In Season
Summer
Autumn
Winter
and Spring

Grows How?
In the ground

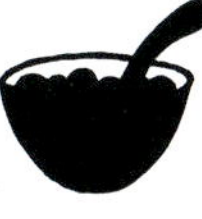

A Serve
1 cup

Good For Your

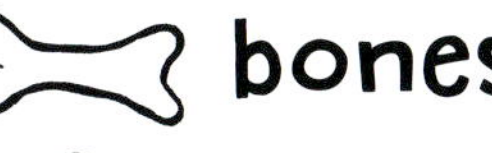

bones
energy

Recipe
Stuffed Mushrooms
(page 50)

BROCCOLI

In Season

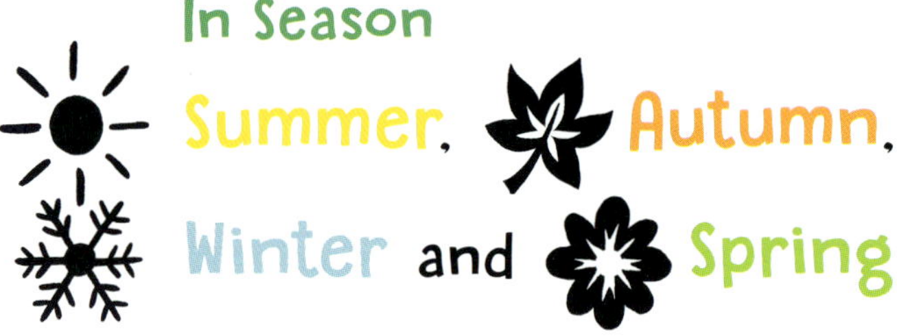

Grows How?

In the ground

A Serve

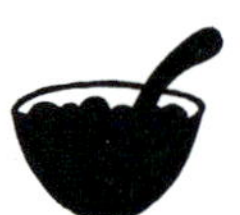
1/2 cup

Good For Your

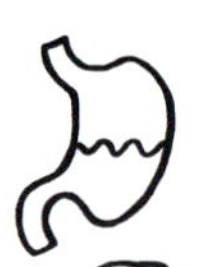
tummy

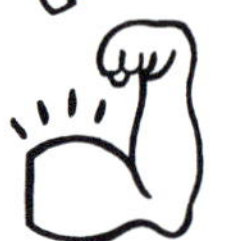
strength

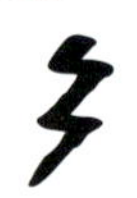
energy

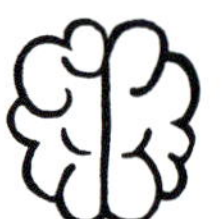
brain

Recipe

Broccoli Noodle Stir Fry (page 42)

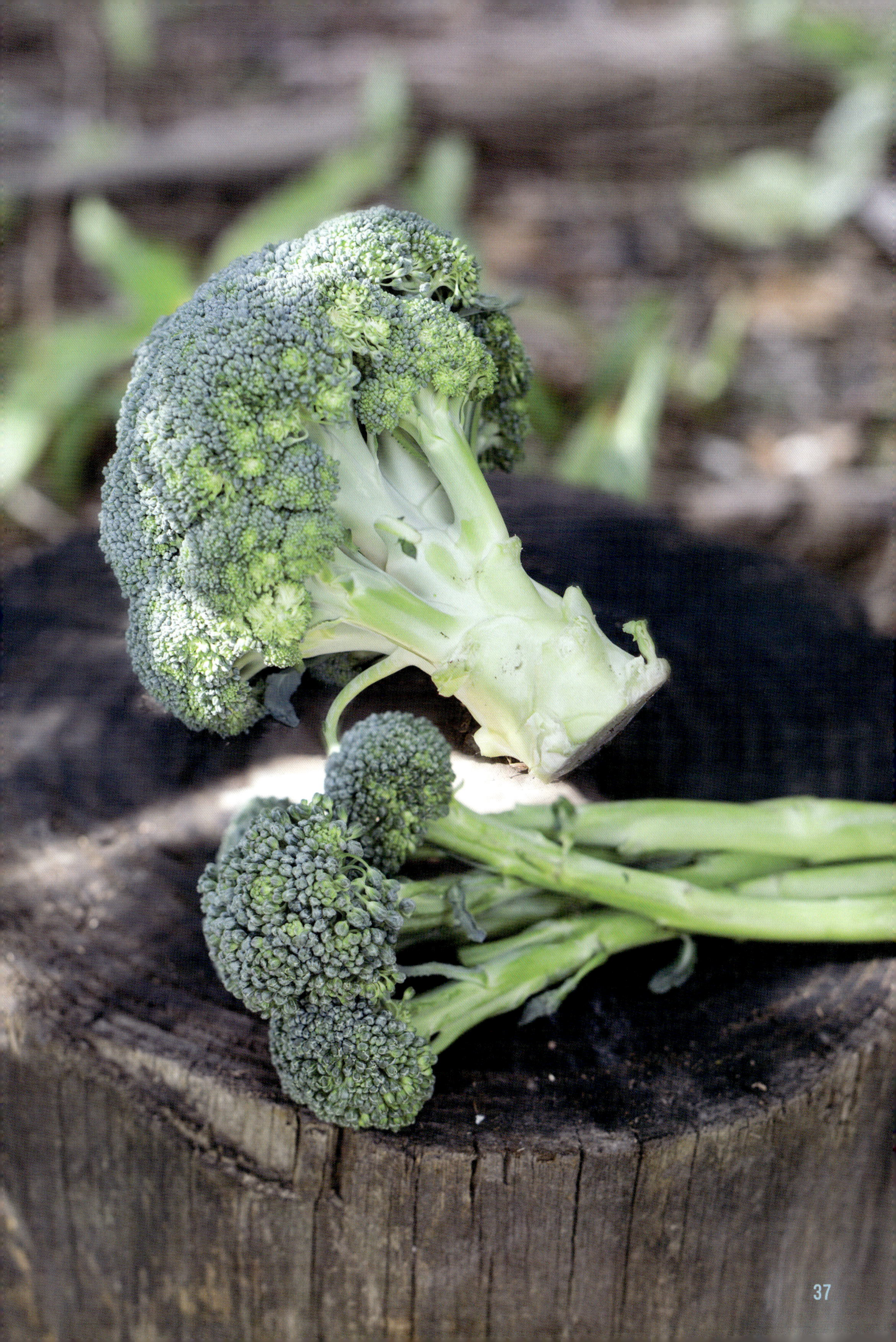

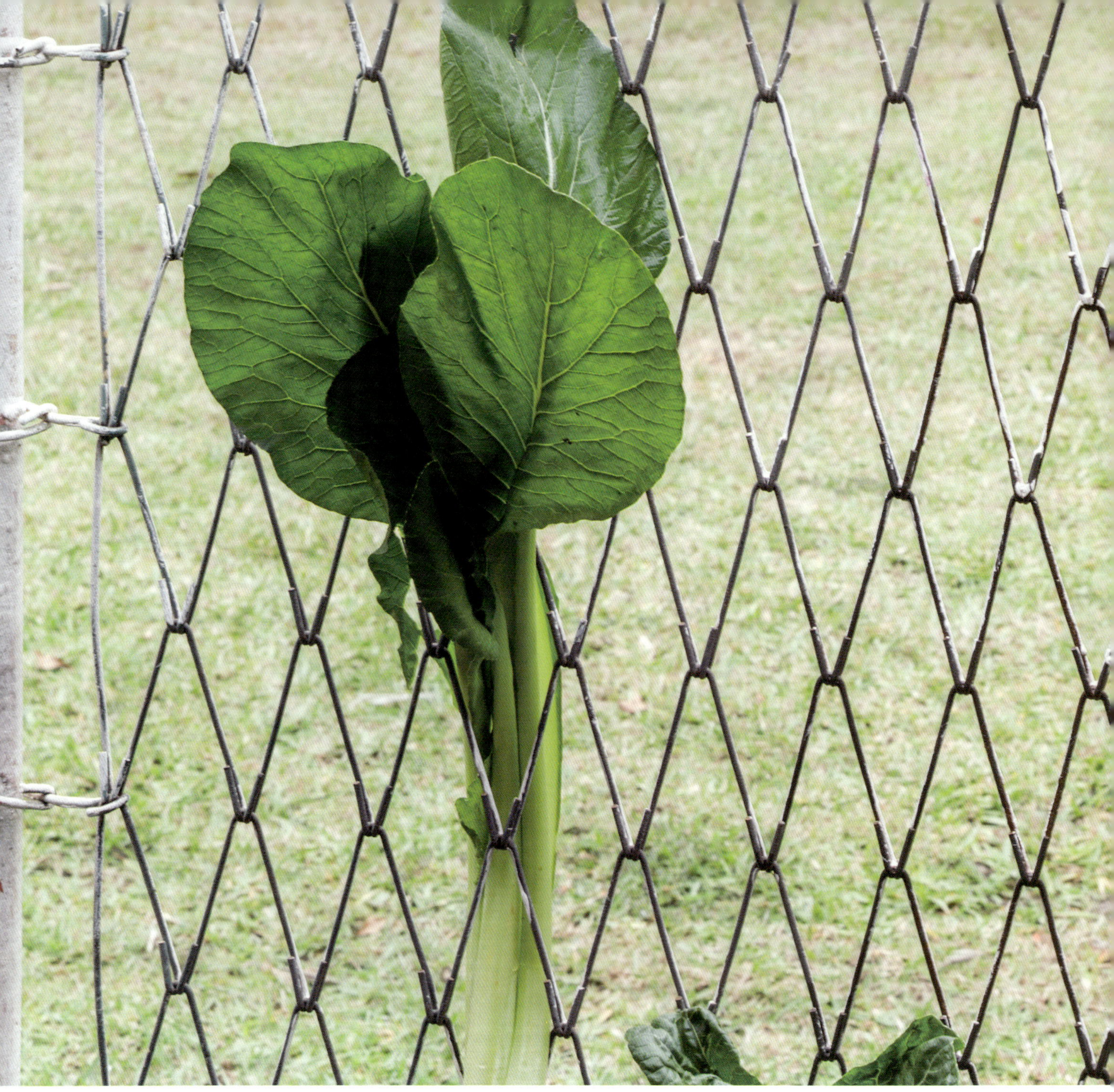

Go to:
www.bitenutrition.com.au
to see the full named picture

ASIAN GREENS

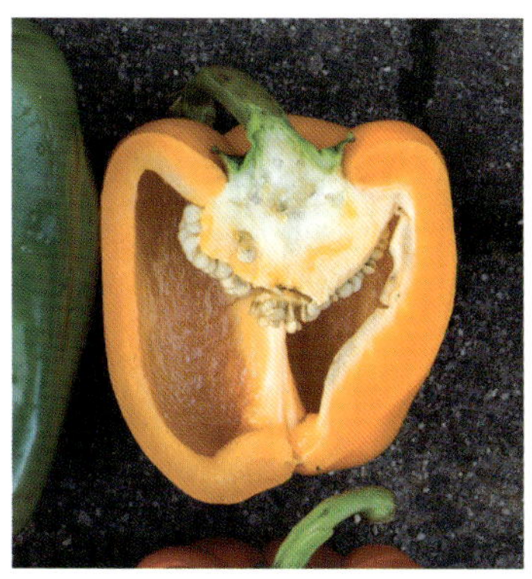

CAPSICUM (page 8)

How to store:

In the fridge in an air tight container.

How to choose:

You want deep color, firm tight skin free of soft spots or blemishes. Heavier the better.

GRILLED CAPSICUM AND BEAN SALAD

- 80g (½ cup) pepitas (pumpkin seed kernels)
- 2 red and 2 yellow capsicums, halved and deseeded, then cut into quarters
- 2 tablespoons olive oil
- 250g green beans, topped
- 100g baby spinach leaves
- 2 tablespoons balsamic vinegar
- 2 tablespoons extra virgin olive oil
- Pinch of sugar
- Freshly ground black pepper

a) Grill the pepitas under the oven griller, on a tray lined with aluminum foil until toasted.

b) Lightly coat (with paper dipped in oil or a baster) capsicums with oil; then grill or chargrill on medium-high for 2-3 minutes on each side until tender and slightly charred. Transfer to a large bowl.

c) Meanwhile, cook the beans in a covered microwave dish with a little water for 2 minutes until tender crisp. Refresh under cold running water. Drain well.

d) Add the pepitas, beans and baby spinach leaves to the capsicums and gently toss until well combined.

e) Whisk together the vinegar, oil and sugar in a small jug until well combined. Taste and season with pepper. Place the salad in a large serving bowl. Drizzle with the dressing and gently toss to combine. Serve immediately.

Serves 4 as a side.

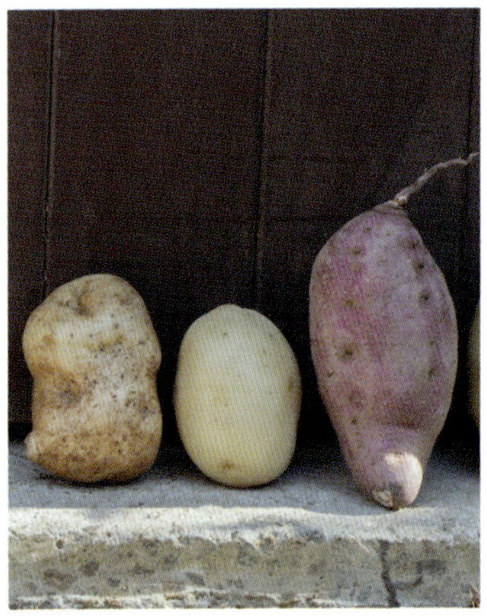

SWEET POTATO AND POTATO (page 32)

How to store:

Store in a cool dark place, not next to onions and not in the fridge. Sweet potatoes last longer if wrapped in newspaper as well.

How to choose:

Smooth and firm without discoloration. No green! No cuts, no bruising, sprouts or soft spots. Sweet potatoes with black ends are starting to go past their due date.

BAKED POTATOES

4 large potatoes, washed and dried

1 can of red kidney beans

1 cup of shredded tasty cheese

2 tomatoes cubed

4 lettuce leaves washed and sliced, or you can also use rocket

1 large grated carrot

1 tsp butter or margarine per potato (½ for cooking and ½ for filling)

Olive oil

Pepper to taste

You can use any potato for baked potato really, but best to use regular unwashed King Edward or Sebago varieties. Our cheat variety of this recipe, for a quick family dinner, is to use the microwave. Prepare the potatoes by pricking them with a fork all over and placing on a plate, cooking on high for around 3-4 minutes per potato (so 12 minutes for 3-4 potatoes). Then cut them open ready for the toppings. If they are still a little hard, just put them back in for a few minutes.

a) Pre heat oven to 200 degrees Celsius.

b) You will need a baking tray and 4 sheets of aluminum foil, large enough to wrap around the potato once.

c) Place ½ teaspoon of butter in the middle of each piece of foil and crack on some pepper. Place one potato per piece of foil, on top of the butter, drizzle with a very small amount of olive oil, then wrap up the potato with the foil.

d) Do this for all the potatoes, then place on baking tray and back for 45 minutes until cooked.

e) Remove from oven and carefully remove the foil (very hot), then cut the potato open in the middle. Put on additional ½ teaspoon of butter and fork the butter through into the potato center.

f) Top each potato with cheese and beans, then place in the microwave for 30 seconds.

g) Then top each potato with remainder of toppings and its ready to serve!